Department of Veterans Affairs
Health Services Research & Development Service | Evidence-based Synthesis Program

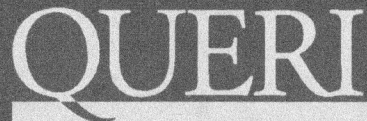

Use of Left Ventricular Assist Devices as Destination Therapy in End-Stage Congestive Heart Failure: A Systematic Review

May 2012

Prepared for:
  Department of Veterans Affairs
  Veterans Health Administration
  Quality Enhancement Research Initiative
  Health Services Research & Development Service
  Washington, DC 20420

Prepared by:
  Evidence-based Synthesis Program (ESP) Center
  Minneapolis VA Medical Center
  Minneapolis, MN
  Timothy J. Wilt, M.D., M.P.H., Director

Investigators:
  Principal Investigators:
    Thomas S. Rector, Ph.D.
    Brent C. Taylor, Ph.D., M.P.H.

  Research Associates:
    Nancy Greer, Ph.D.
    Indulis Rutks, B.S.

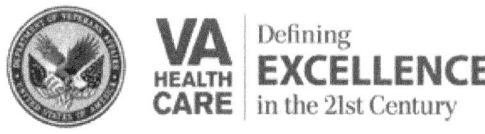

PREFACE

Quality Enhancement Research Initiative's (QUERI) Evidence-based Synthesis Program (ESP) was established to provide timely and accurate syntheses of targeted healthcare topics of particular importance to Veterans Affairs (VA) managers and policymakers, as they work to improve the health and healthcare of Veterans. The ESP disseminates these reports throughout VA.

QUERI provides funding for four ESP Centers and each Center has an active VA affiliation. The ESP Centers generate evidence syntheses on important clinical practice topics, and these reports help:
- develop clinical policies informed by evidence,
- guide the implementation of effective services to improve patient outcomes and to support VA clinical practice guidelines and performance measures, and
- set the direction for future research to address gaps in clinical knowledge.

In 2009, the ESP Coordinating Center was created to expand the capacity of QUERI Central Office and the four ESP sites by developing and maintaining program processes. In addition, the Center established a Steering Committee comprised of QUERI field-based investigators, VA Patient Care Services, Office of Quality and Performance, and Veterans Integrated Service Networks (VISN) Clinical Management Officers. The Steering Committee provides program oversight, guides strategic planning, coordinates dissemination activities, and develops collaborations with VA leadership to identify new ESP topics of importance to Veterans and the VA healthcare system.

Comments on this evidence report are welcome and can be sent to Nicole Floyd, ESP Coordinating Center Program Manager, at nicole.floyd@va.gov.

Recommended citation: Rector TS, Taylor BC, Greer N, Rutks I, and Wilt TJ. Use of Left Ventricular Assist Devices as Destination Therapy in End-Stage Congestive Heart Failure: A Systematic Review. VA-ESP Project #09-009; 2012.

This report is based on research conducted by the Evidence-based Synthesis Program (ESP) Center located at the Minneapolis VA Medical Center, Minneapolis, MN funded by the Department of Veterans Affairs, Veterans Health Administration, Office of Research and Development, Quality Enhancement Research Initiative. The findings and conclusions in this document are those of the author(s) who are responsible for its contents; the findings and conclusions do not necessarily represent the views of the Department of Veterans Affairs or the United States government. Therefore, no statement in this article should be construed as an official position of the Department of Veterans Affairs. No investigators have any affiliations or financial involvement (e.g., employment, consultancies, honoraria, stock ownership or options, expert testimony, grants or patents received or pending, or royalties) that conflict with material presented in the report.

TABLE OF CONTENTS

EXECUTIVE SUMMARY
Background 1
Methods 1
Data Synthesis 2
Peer Review 2
Results 2
Recommendations for Future Research 4

INTRODUCTION 5
Ventricular Assist Devices Approved for Use as Destination Therapy 6
Centers for Medicare and Medicaid Services (CMS) Coverage 6
Registry of Ventricular Assist Devices Used as Destination Therapy 7
Guideline Recommendations 7

METHODS
Topic Development 9
Search Strategy 9
Study Selection 10
Data Abstraction 12
Quality Assessment 12
Rating the Body of Evidence 13
Data Synthesis 14
Peer Review 14

RESULTS
Literature Search 15
Key Question #1. How does use of an FDA-approved, current generation LVAD as destination therapy (i.e., the HeartMate II left ventricular assist device) effect patient outcomes? 15
Key Question #2. What patient or site characteristics have been associated with patient benefits or harms when the FDA-approved, current generation LVAD is used as destination therapy? 17
Key Question #3. What is the range of cost-effectiveness estimates of using the FDA-approved, current generation LVAD as destination therapy in end-stage heart failure and what explains variation in these estimates? 19

SUMMARY AND DISCUSSION
Summary Points 21
Limitations 21
Recommendations for Future Research 21
Conclusions 23

REFERENCES 24

FIGURES

Figure 1. Analytic Framework 10

Figure 2. Literature Flow Diagram 15

APPENDIX A. TECHNICAL EXPERT PANEL MEMBERS 27

APPENDIX B. SEARCH STRATEGY 28

APPENDIX C. PEER REVIEW COMMENTS/AUTHOR RESPONSES 29

APPENDIX D. EVIDENCE TABLES

Table 1. Key Question #1: Effects on Patient Outcomes 34

Table 2. Key Question #2: Patient Selection 38

Table 3. Key Question #3: Cost-effectiveness 41

EXECUTIVE SUMMARY

BACKGROUND

Heart failure is defined as reduced ability of the heart to pump blood and maintain normal bodily function. Heart transplantation is currently the preferred treatment for end-stage heart failure but the supply of donor hearts is insufficient to meet the need and many patients are not eligible for transplantation due to age or comorbid conditions.

Implantable mechanical pumps can assist the circulation of blood by the ventricles. Left ventricular assist devices (LVADs) have been approved by the U.S. Food and Drug Administration (FDA) for use in patients awaiting transplant (a bridge to transplant) and as a last resort in patients with refractory heart failure who are not eligible for a heart transplant (destination therapy). In January 2010, the first newer generation, rotary continuous flow ventricular assist device (HeartMate II) was approved by the FDA for destination therapy. Eligibility criteria are essentially the same as those used to select patients for the pivotal clinical trial that included patients with shortness of breath and/or fatigue at rest or during minimal exertion despite treatment with optimal therapy for heart failure associated with a low ejection fraction (< 25%) who were not candidates for heart transplantation due to their age or co-morbid conditions. The purpose of this report is to review the scientific evidence for use of the current generation of left ventricular assist devices as destination therapy.

The key questions were:

Key Question #1. How does use of an FDA-approved, current generation LVAD as destination therapy (i.e., the HeartMate II left ventricular assist device) effect patient outcomes?

Key Question #2. What patient or site characteristics have been associated with patient benefits or harms when the FDA-approved, current generation LVAD is used as destination therapy?

Key Question #3. What is the range of cost-effectiveness estimates of using the FDA-approved, current generation LVAD as destination therapy in end-stage heart failure and what explains variation in these estimates?

METHODS

We searched MEDLINE using standard search terms (Appendix B). The search was limited to articles involving human subjects and published in the English language from 1995 to October 2011. We also searched the Cochrane Database of Systematic Reviews, the Translating Research into Practice (TRIP) database for systematic reviews and technology assessments, the Center for Medicare and Medicaid Services (CMS) Web site and the NIH Clinical Trials Web site. Reference lists of articles and reports were reviewed to identify additional references. Information was extracted from eligible articles by the investigators. Study quality was assessed using criteria appropriate for the design of the studies identified to address the three key questions (comparison studies, prognostic studies or cost-effectiveness analyses).

DATA SYNTHESIS

Evidence tables were constructed for each key question to summarize each study included in the review including patient and intervention characteristics, patient outcomes (benefits and harms) and methodological quality. Qualitative syntheses of the available data were done to answer each of the 3 key questions. There were not enough similar studies to pool data using formal meta-analysis in an effort to get more precise estimates. Any findings, or lack thereof, representing the Departments of Veterans Affairs or Defense (DoD) populations were noted.

PEER REVIEW

A draft version of this report was reviewed by the technical expert panel, as well as other expert health care providers. Reviewer comments and our responses are summarized in Appendix C.

RESULTS

The electronic search identified 1,637 citations. Preliminary review of the titles and abstracts excluded 1,491 from further review; 146 were retained for more in-depth review. From these, we identified 3 articles for Key Question #1, 3 articles for Key Question #2 and no articles for Key Question #3. A search of reference lists and identification of recently published studies added one article for each key question.

Key Question #1. How does use of an FDA-approved, current generation LVAD as destination therapy (i.e., the HeartMate II left ventricular assist device) effect patient outcomes?

Conclusion

- A single study provides moderate strength evidence that use of the HeartMate II as a destination left ventricular assist device produces better patient outcomes, including patient survival, with fewer harms and hospitalizations than the HeartMate XVE, the only other ventricular assist device approved by the FDA for destination therapy.

We found one good quality randomized clinical trial of the HeartMate II used as a left ventricular assist device for destination therapy.[1] Patients enrolled in this study met the general criteria for destination therapy that were largely based on enrollment criteria in a previous study of an older generation device[2] including being ineligible for a heart transplant, being symptomatic at rest or with minimal exertion (New York Heart Association [NYHA] class IV heart failure) despite optimization of other therapies for heart failure, and a left ventricular ejection fraction less than 25%. Thus the findings are likely applicable to current candidates for destination therapy. The subjects' (n=200) mean age was 62 years and 84% were male. Compared to the older generation HeartMate XVE left ventricular assist device, use of the HeartMate II had better patient outcomes (See Appendix D, Table 1). After 24 months, the primary endpoint of survival free of disabling stroke or reoperation to remove the device was 46% versus 11% (p < 0.0001). Survival in the HeartMate II group was significantly better (58% versus 24% after 2 years) and subjects spent a greater percentage of their follow-up time outside of a hospital (88% versus 74%) largely due to a lower readmission rate. During follow-up survivors with the HeartMate II also had fewer functional limitations due to heart failure as measured by the NYHA class, Minnesota Living with Heart Failure Questionnaire and clinical component of the Kansas City Cardiomyopathy Questionnaire. The incidences of several adverse events were lower as well including right heart failure, cardiac arrhythmias, device-related infections, sepsis, respiratory failure, renal failure, and device replacement. None of the adverse events rates were higher in the HeartMate II group than the HeartMate XVE group including major bleeding and strokes.

Currently all cases of destination therapy being registered in a national data base are being treated with the HeartMate II device.[3] Since patient characteristics and outcomes in the HeartMate XVE arm of this randomized comparison of devices were similar to those in the previous clinical trial that demonstrated the HeartMate VE provided superior outcomes compared to optimal medical therapy,[2] one might infer that the HeartMate II would also be superior to optimal medical therapy. Clinical trials of other newer generation continuous flow ventricular assist devices for destination therapy are ongoing, however, results are not expected for several years.

Key Question #2. What patient or site characteristics have been associated with patient benefits or harms when the FDA-approved, current generation LVAD is used as destination therapy?

Conclusion

- The available evidence is insufficient to refine patient or site selection criteria for use of the HeartMate II as destination therapy.

A few studies have identified risk factors for mortality and complications and developed or applied mortality prediction models to this particular patient population. Further studies are needed to validate use of different criteria to improve patient outcomes. An ongoing clinical trial is selecting less severely ill patients and may expand the criteria for use of a newer generation continuous flow device (HeartWare) as destination therapy.[4,5] In the meantime, the approved FDA indication and CMS criteria for coverage are available to guide patient selection.

Key Question #3. What is the range of cost-effectiveness estimates of using the FDA-approved, current generation LVAD as destination therapy in end-stage heart failure and what explains variation in these estimates?

Conclusion

- A single industry funded analysis has estimated that the cost-effectiveness of using the FDA-approved, current generation LVAD as destination therapy in patients with end-stage heart disease is approximately $200,000 per quality-adjusted life year. The strength of the evidence for this estimate is low.

Even with favorable assumptions regarding the cost and effectiveness of treatment, destination therapy using the current generation, continuous flow ventricular assist device appears to be relatively cost-ineffective compared with traditional standards and other Medicare approved interventions.[6] However, large improvements in cost-effectiveness have occurred in the past decade. If improvements continue to be made, destination therapy in end-stage heart disease with an LVAD may become more cost-effective in the future.

RECOMMENDATIONS FOR FUTURE RESEARCH

Additional high-quality data are needed to inform clinical practices and policies regarding the use of ventricular assist devices to treat patients with end-stage heart failure who are not eligible for a heart transplant. Investigators suggest the following recommendations regarding future research:

- Create or participate in a registry of all Veterans that receive an LVAD as destination therapy, and support enrollment of Veterans in ongoing, randomized controlled clinical trials.

- Develop decision aids to help providers communicate information about the benefits, risks and care needed when patients are considering an approved ventricular assist device as destination therapy and to help providers elicit patients' values and preferences.

- Update cost-effectiveness models as better data become available and incorporate probabilistic sensitivity analyses to assess uncertainty in the cost-effectiveness estimates.

- Conduct a budget impact analysis that specifically addresses the potential impact within the Veterans Health Administration of use of the currently approved continuous flow ventricular assist devices as destination therapy.

EVIDENCE REPORT

INTRODUCTION

Several common chronic conditions such as atherosclerotic heart disease and hypertension as well as other diseases can result in heart failure, a reduced ability of the heart to pump blood and maintain normal bodily functions. The prevalence of chronic heart failure increases with age to over 10% in the elderly population.[7] More than 100,000 people in the United States with progressive heart failure are refractory to available treatments and have high rates of hospitalization and mortality and a poor quality of life due to limited physical and social activities and psychological stress. Heart transplantation is currently the preferred treatment for end-stage heart failure. Unfortunately, the supply of donor hearts is far less than needed and many patients do not meet the criteria for heart transplantation primarily due to old age and comorbidities such as diabetes with damage to vital organs, pulmonary hypertension, renal insufficiency, malignancies and morbid obesity.

Implantable mechanical pumps that assist the circulation of blood by one or both ventricles of the heart have evolved over several decades. Typically blood flows from the native left ventricle of the heart into the surgically implanted assist device and is pumped out into the aorta via an implanted conduit. The design of the mechanical pump varies (pulsatile fill and pump designs similar to a normal heart and continuous flow rotary pumps). Currently, long-term implantable left ventricular assist devices require an external source of power and control module.

Surgical placement of a left ventricular assist device is increasingly done as a last resort for patients with refractory heart failure who are not eligible for heart transplantation, so called destination therapy.[8] Some patients may improve after they receive a ventricular assist device as destination therapy and become eligible for heart transplantation even though this was not the initial therapeutic goal. A limited number may recover enough heart function to not need a heart transplant or mechanical assist device. Although survival with a newer generation continuous flow ventricular assist device is approaching that of a heart transplant, long-term use of the device by patients who are eligible for a heart transplant is not currently accepted practice.[9] Conversely, many patients that receive a ventricular assist device as a bridge to transplant use the device for increasingly prolonged periods while waiting for a donated heart and some may become ineligible for a heart transplant.

The purpose of this report is to review the scientific evidence for use of ventricular assist devices as destination therapy for patients with severe, refractory heart failure who are not eligible for heart transplantation at the time the device is implanted. Although many patients receive the same types of ventricular assist devices as a bridge to heart transplantation or recovery, the characteristics, hence risk profiles, of patients receiving bridge therapy are different from patients selected to receive a device as permanent destination therapy. Furthermore many bridged patients do receive a heart transplant that alters patient outcomes. Thus, this review focused on evidence about patient outcomes, patient selection and cost effectiveness of ventricular assist devices specifically intended as destination therapy. The primary goals of destination therapy are to:

- prolong survival,
- improve daily function and health-related quality of life,
- minimize harms including infection, major bleeding episodes, thromboembolic events including strokes and device malfunction or failure especially those that require hospital care.

VENTRICULAR ASSIST DEVICES APPROVED FOR USE AS DESTINATION THERAPY

The first randomized controlled clinical trial of a ventricular assist device as destination therapy compared an early generation device (a ventilated electric pulsatile pump, HeartMate VE) to optimal medical therapy.[2] This device significantly improved survival to 52% versus 25% at 1 year and 23% versus 8% after 2 years. Unfortunately, 35% of the surgically implanted devices failed within 2 years, and 17% of the deaths were attributed to failure of the device. The overall effect of the device, including serious complications on the subjects' functional status and health-related quality of life, was difficult to assess due to the high, differential mortality rates and lack of assessments during early follow-up. Comparisons of the subjects that survived for one year indicated physical and emotional status were better in the group treated with the ventricular assist device. This pivotal trial led to approval by the U.S. Food and Drug Administration (FDA) in November 2002 of the left ventricular assist device (modified and now known as the HeartMate XVE) for use as destination therapy.[10] The approved indication included patients that were not eligible for heart transplantation who have New York Heart Association (NYHA) class IV heart failure (shortness of breath and/or fatigue during minimal physical activity or at rest) for at least 60 of the last 90 days despite optimal medical therapy, an unassisted left ventricular ejection fraction less than 25%, and a peak oxygen consumption less than 12 ml/kg/min during an exercise stress test or continued need for an intravenous inotrope. Furthermore, the estimated life expectancy without the ventricular assist device should be less than 2 years, similar to patients that participated in the clinical trial. After FDA approval, clinical use of the HeartMate XVE was associated with a similar 56% 1-year survival, but unfavorable rates of surgical complications including sepsis, multi-organ failure, right heart failure, prolonged hospitalization and a 90-day in-hospital mortality of 27%.[11] Within 2 years, 73% needed device replacement or experienced a fatal device failure.

In January 2010, a newer generation, rotary continuous flow ventricular assist device (HeartMate II) was approved by the FDA for destination therapy based on a clinical trial that compared the new ventricular assist device, the HeartMate II, to the HeartMate XVE.

CENTERS FOR MEDICARE AND MEDICAID SERVICES (CMS) COVERAGE

In October 2003, the Centers for Medicare and Medicaid Services (CMS) decided to cover use of FDA-approved ventricular assist devices as destination therapy when provided by a Medicare-approved heart transplantation center.[12] The clinical center needed to have the staff and processes to fully inform prospective recipients about the potential benefits, risks and required follow-up care. Furthermore, the center was required to report case information to a national audited registry from the date of device implantation until death. In March 2007, the facility criteria were modified to require a board-certified cardiovascular surgeon that has implanted at least 10 ventricular assist devices during the past 3 years (at least one in past 18 months) and facility certification by the Disease-Specific Care Certification Program for Ventricular Assist Device developed by the Joint Commission on Accreditation of Healthcare Organizations.

After FDA approval of the HeartMate II device for destination therapy, CMS eligibility requirements were changed to include patients that are refractory to optimal medical management for at least 45 of the past 60 days or dependent on an intra-aortic balloon pump for 7 days or an intravenous inotrope for 14 days. The peak oxygen requirement was increased to 14 ml/kg/min or less unless the patient was physically unable to do an exercise test or was dependent on a balloon pump or intravenous inotrope.

REGISTRY OF VENTRICULAR ASSIST DEVICES USED AS DESTINATION THERAPY

An Interagency Registry for Mechanically Assisted Circulatory Support (INTERMACS) was created with support from the National Heart, Lung and Blood Institute, FDA, CMS, the device industry and health care providers. In June 2006, this registry began to collect information about patients, devices and outcomes including adverse events. The registry is focused on use of FDA-approved ventricular assist devices including destination therapy. The registry meets the CMS mandate that all hospitals in the United States that provide mechanical circulatory support as destination therapy enter their cases into a national audited registry.[3] During the 6-month period from January to June 2010 (shortly after FDA approval of the new continuous flow device, HeartMate II), there was nearly a 10-fold increase in the number of registered uses for destination therapy. All registered cases during this period received the newer FDA-approved HeartMate II ventricular assist device. As of June 30, 2011, 126 medical centers had registered patients of which 101 centers were approved by CMS to provide destination therapy.[13] A total of 847 patients treated with destination therapy had been registered and all recent cases employed the FDA approved continuous flow ventricular assist device, presumably HeartMate II. *No VA Medical Centers were listed by the registry as of March 5, 2012 (see www.intermacs. org/membership).* Patients receiving a continuous device as destination therapy had significantly worse survival than those receiving a continuous device as a bridge to transplant.

GUIDELINE RECOMMENDATIONS

A 2009 update of the 2005 American College of Cardiology Foundation/American Heart Association Task Force on Practice Guidelines for the Diagnosis and Management of Heart Failure in Adults did not modify their previous recommendation concerning destination therapy for patients with refractory end-stage heart failure (stage D).[14] Consideration of a permanent left ventricular assist device continued to be considered reasonable for highly selected (undefined) patients that have estimated 1-year mortality with optimal medical therapy over 50%. This recommendation was developed in collaboration with International Society for Heart Lung Transplantation.

Guidelines issued by the Heart Failure Society of America in 2010 recommend that permanent mechanical assistance may be considered in highly selected patients with severe heart failure refractory to conventional therapy who are not candidates for heart transplantation, particularly those who cannot be weaned from inotropic support by an experienced heart failure center.[15]

The 2011 Canadian Cardiovascular Society Heart Failure Guidelines recommend that permanent mechanical circulatory support be considered for highly selected patients who are ineligible for heart transplantation.[16] This was considered to be a 'weak' recommendation because of the uncertainty about the balance of benefits and risk given currently available evidence. Eligible candidates would have severe symptoms of advanced heart failure despite optimal treatment and meet at least two of the following criteria: 1) a left ventricle ejection fraction less than 25% and, if exercise stress test is done, a peak oxygen consumption less than 14 ml/kg/min, 2) progressive organ dysfunction due to hypoperfusion, 3) need to reduce standard therapies for heart failure due to symptomatic hypotension or worsening renal function, 4) more than 3 hospital admissions for refractory heart failure during the previous year or 5) unable to wean from inotropic support. Informed patient preferences were a very important component of the recommendation as was a medical center that has a multidisciplinary team with expertise in surgical implantation and follow-up of patients with ventricular assist devices.

METHODS

TOPIC DEVELOPMENT

This project was nominated by Dr. Chester Good, Chief, Section of General Medicine. The key questions were developed with input from a technical expert panel (see Appendix A).

The final key questions were:

Key Question #1. How does use of an FDA-approved, current generation LVAD as destination therapy (i.e., the HeartMate II left ventricular assist device) effect patient outcomes?

Key Question #2. What patient or site characteristics have been associated with patient benefits or harms when the FDA-approved, current generation LVAD is used as destination therapy?

Key Question #3. What is the range of cost-effectiveness estimates of using the FDA-approved, current generation LVAD as destination therapy in end-stage heart failure and what explains variation in these estimates?

Figure 1 depicts the analytic framework for these questions.

SEARCH STRATEGY

We searched MEDLINE (OVID) for studies that reported patient outcomes, articles about patient selection or prediction of patient outcomes, systematic reviews or cost-effectiveness analyses from 1995 to October 2011 using standard search terms. The 1995 start date is well before the first randomized clinical trial that used a left ventricular assist device for destination therapy. The search was limited to articles involving human subjects and published in the English language. Search terms included: heart-assist devices, heart failure and ventricular dysfunction (See Appendix B for the MEDLINE search strategy). We also examined reference lists to identify other pertinent publications and asked our panel of experts to identify additional reports.

Other searches included the Cochrane Database of Systematic Reviews, the Translating Research into Practice (TRIP) database for systematic reviews and technology assessments, the Center for Medicare and Medicaid Services (CMS) Web site and the NIH Clinical Trials Web site.

Figure 1. Analytic Framework

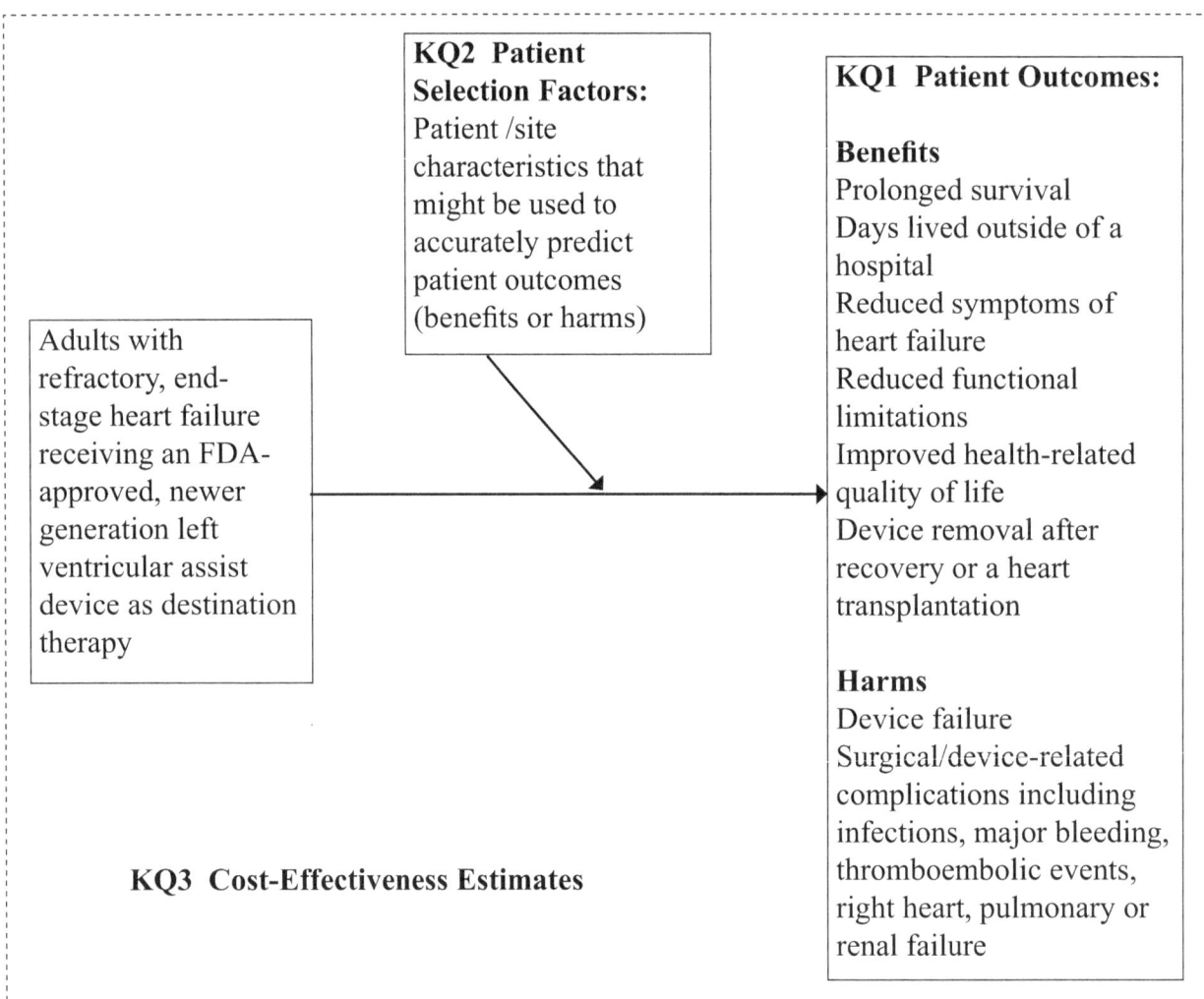

STUDY SELECTION

Generally, abstracts and full text articles were excluded whenever

1. The report did not provide data about the only continuous flow device currently approved by FDA for destination therapy, the HeartMate II ventricular assist device.
2. The report did not provide data about use of the device as destination therapy. Short-term use of the device as a bridge to transplant was excluded.
3. The report did not provide data about patient outcomes of interest such as survival, hospitalizations, daily function, health-related quality of life or harms.
4. The report did not provide data about adults defined as age 18 years or older.

The following discusses more specific study selection criteria for each key question.

Key Question #1 – Patient Outcomes

Randomized controlled trials were sought as the highest quality of evidence for the first key question about patient outcomes. At a minimum, randomization helps assure unbiased allocation of subjects to the groups being compared. However, the number of patients currently eligible for destination device therapy is limited and randomization might not balance baseline characteristics in small studies. Subjects that withdraw from the study after randomization or crossover to the comparison group may also bias the comparison, particularly if any changes in treatment were related to study outcomes. Obviously a comparison of a surgically implanted device to continuation of optimal medical therapy can't be blinded, and endpoint assessments, especially subjective assessments and device-related harms, may be biased as a result. However, more objective endpoints such as maximal exercise tests are affected by patient effort and difficult to interpret in terms of how they translate into affects on patients' lives. Given the high morbidity and mortality of patients with refractory end-stage heart failure, randomization to continuation of non-surgical therapies might not be acceptable to patients and providers who believe a ventricular assist device is a reasonable alternative. Therefore, randomized clinical trials are being designed as a non-inferiority comparison of a new ventricular assist device to an approved device.[17,18] Non-inferiority studies introduce additional concerns that the characteristics of the enrolled subjects, including how they were treated, might not be similar to previous studies that demonstrated the 'control' device is effective with acceptable risks.[19] Furthermore, the magnitude of the differences between devices excluded by the statistical analysis of non-inferiority needs to be small enough to rule out clinically important differences. Since high quality evidence from randomized clinical trials of the FDA-approved continuous flow ventricular assist device for destination therapy is very limited, we did not restrict our review to randomized controlled trials, and considered cohort studies that could provide estimates of the likelihood of patient outcomes.

Key Question #2 – Patient Selection

Given numerous differences in outcomes including device malfunction between the two ventricular assist devices currently approved for use as destination therapy, the HeartMate XVE and HeartMate II, and the current exclusive use of the HeartMate II device for destination therapy in the INTERMACS registry, our search for the second key question concerning selection of patients sought specific analyses about the HeartMate II ventricular assist device. As previously mentioned, we also focused on selection of patients for destination therapy rather than bridge therapy because the criteria and outcomes including competing risks such as heart transplantation are not the same. Thus, studies were selected if they provided evidence specifically or predominantly about the selection of patients for use of the HeartMate II device as destination therapy. Subgroup analyses that focused on this specific therapy were considered including regression analysis that included variables indicating the type of ventricular assist device and/or therapy.

Patient selection criteria for destination therapy are based primarily on the selection criteria used in the studies that supported FDA approval and therefore define patients eligible for the approved indication. However, regression or subgroup analyses are often conducted using study data or other patient cohorts in an effort to better define which patients are more likely to benefit or be harmed. Studies were sought that provided statistical evidence for significant differences in patient outcomes between groups defined by preoperative patient characteristics. Expert reviews of patient selection criteria were read in search of additional scientific evidence about patient selection criteria. Because estimates of patient survival without the ventricular assist device are used to select patients, we also included studies that evaluated survival prediction models in a sample of patients eligible for destination therapy.

Key Question #3 – Cost Effectiveness

We included studies that provided cost-effectiveness estimates for the use of HeartMate II ventricular assist device as destination therapy.

DATA ABSTRACTION

For reports that provided pertinent evidence about patient outcomes and selection (Key Questions #1 and #2), we extracted information about the study sites and sponsor, subject inclusion and exclusion criteria, sample characteristics, intervention(s) including the comparison group(s), if any, length of follow-up, patient outcome(s) of interest and quality of the evidence.

For reports that provided pertinent evidence about cost effectiveness (Key Question #3), we extracted information about the overall estimate of cost effectiveness, the uncertainty in the cost effectiveness estimate, the base case assumptions for the cost effectiveness model and the results of sensitivity analyses that varied the assumptions in the base case model.

QUALITY ASSESSMENT

Key Question #1 – Patient Outcomes

The quality of clinical trials was judged based on the potential for bias in the estimates of treatment effects according to the following criteria: 1) random assignment to treatment with adequate concealment of assignment, 2) blinding of key study personnel (i.e., providers, study personnel and/or patients) who determined outcomes to assigned treatment, 3) analysis by intention-to-treat (i.e., all subjects counted in group to which they were randomized in the analysis of outcomes), 4) reporting of number of withdrawals/dropouts by group assignment along with reasons for any losses to follow-up that may be related to beneficial or adverse treatment effects and 5) the size of the treatment effects (larger effects are less likely to be explained by baseline differences between treatment groups or differential losses to follow-up).[20] Studies were rated as good, fair, or poor quality. A rating of 'good quality' generally required that the investigators randomly assigned patients to treatments and reported adequate concealment of assignments, blinded or objective outcome assessments, an intent-to-treat analysis, an adequate description of reasons for dropouts/attrition and a sizable treatment effect. The quality of a study was generally considered poor if the method of allocation concealment was inadequate or not defined, blinding was not reported or possible, analysis by intent-to-treat was not reported and reasons for dropouts/attrition were not reported and/or there was a high rate of attrition or the estimated treatment effect was small.

Key Question #2 – Patient Selection

Criteria to assess the quality of evidence concerning variables and multivariable models to predict patient outcomes have not been firmly established. We relied on our, as yet unpublished, guidance for conducting systematic reviews of prognostic tests commissioned by the Agency for Healthcare Research and Quality (Rector TS, Taylor BG, Wilt TJ. Chapter 12: Systematic Reviews of Prognostic Tests in *Methods Guide for Comparative Effectiveness Reviews*). Specific criteria: 1) were patients in the analysis similar to those who would receive an FDA-approved ventricular assist device as destination therapy?, 2) were the variables used to make outcome predictions measured shortly before implantation of the device and not affected by the procedure, subsequent care or knowledge of the outcome being predicted?, 3) were the measurements of the potential predictor variables and outcomes reliable, valid and routinely available in clinical practice?, 4) did losses to follow-up bias the assessment of outcomes?, 5) was the duration of follow-up adequate?, 6) were the number of patients that had the outcome being predicted adequate for the number of predictors tested?, 7) were predicted outcome probabilities reported for patient subgroups that would be included or excluded from destination therapy?, 8) how closely did outcome predictions agree with the observed outcomes?, 9) were the outcome prediction somehow validated? and 10) did the analysis demonstrate that the outcome predictions could be used to improve patient outcomes?

Key Question #3 – Cost Effectiveness

There are no well-accepted criteria for evaluating the quality of cost-effectiveness analyses, however, there are long lists of factors related to the analytical model and assumptions that can be considered.[21] In order to assess quality we extracted information on the cost-effectiveness model structure and assumptions.

RATING THE BODY OF EVIDENCE

The overall evidence for a key question was graded using the method proposed by Owens et al.[23] using the following criteria:

- High grade evidence: Further research is very unlikely to change the confidence in the estimated treatment effect on patient outcomes. Generally, a high grade requires more than one good quality study and consistent estimates with statistical confidence intervals that exclude clinically meaningful differences.

- Moderate grade evidence: Further research may change the estimate of the size of the effect or the level of uncertainty.

- Low grade evidence: Further research is likely to change the estimate of the size of the effect and or the confidence interval.

- Insufficient evidence: Sufficient evidence was not found to answer the question.

DATA SYNTHESIS

We constructed evidence tables for Key Questions #1, #2 and #3, and drew our conclusions based on a qualitative synthesis of the evidence available to answer each key question. Not finding several reports that provided independent estimates of patient outcomes, relationships between baseline variables and patient outcomes or cost effectiveness, we did not do any meta-analyses to pool evidence from different studies.

PEER REVIEW

A draft version of this report was reviewed by clinical experts including the Technical Expert Panel. Their comments are presented in Appendix C as are our responses to any suggestions to modify the report itself.

RESULTS

LITERATURE SEARCH

Figure 2 summarizes the literature search. We reviewed 1,637 titles and abstracts from the electronic search. After applying inclusion/exclusion criteria, 1,491 references were excluded. We retrieved 146 full-text articles for further review and 140 were excluded. We identified 1 additional reference by hand-searching references lists and 2 articles that were published after our search date. There were a total of 4 articles (3 from the literature search) for Key Question #1; only one was a randomized controlled trial. There were 4 articles included for Key Question #2 (3 from the literature search); 3 examined prediction models and 1 was a subgroup analysis. For Key Question #3, 1 article was included that was published after the initial literature search.

Figure 2. Literature Flow Diagram

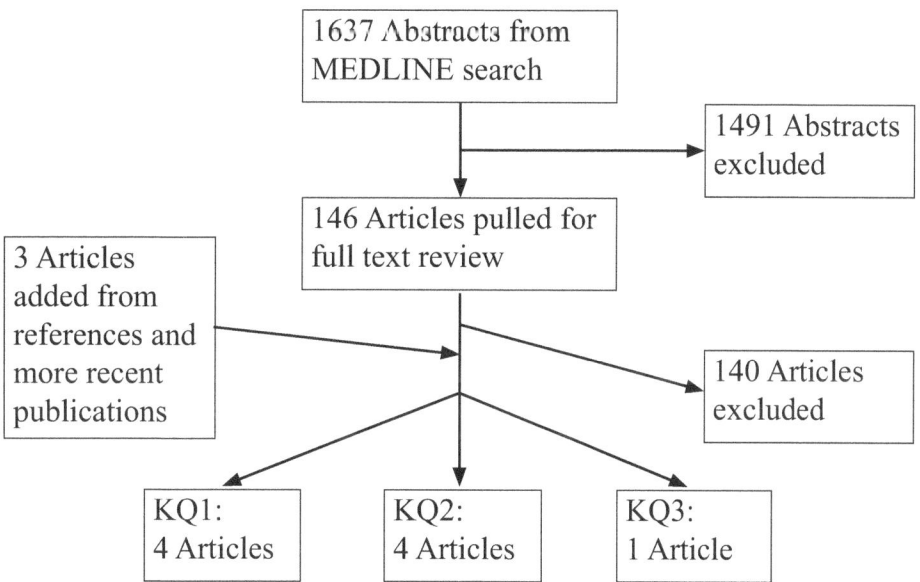

KEY QUESTION #1. How does use of an FDA-approved, current generation LVAD as destination therapy (i.e., the HeartMate II left ventricular assist device) effect patient outcomes?

We found one good quality randomized clinical trial of the HeartMate II left ventricular assist device employed as destination therapy.[1] Patients enrolled in this study generally met the current criteria for destination therapy that were based on a previous study of an older generation device[2] including being ineligible for a heart transplant, most being in NYHA association class IV heart failure that was refractory to optimized therapies, a left ventricular ejection fraction less than 25% and very limited ability to exercise. The subjects' (n=200) mean age was 62 years and 84% were males. Compared to the older generation HeartMate XVE left ventricular assist device, use of the HeartMate II provided superior patient outcomes (See Appendix D, Table 1). After 24 months, the primary endpoint of survival free of disabling stroke or reoperation to remove the device was 46% versus 11%, respectively (p < 0.0001). Survival in the HeartMate II group was significantly better (58% versus 24% after 2 years) and subjects spent a greater percentage of their follow-up time outside of a hospital (88% versus 74%) largely due to a lower readmission rate. During follow-up, survivors with the HeartMate II also had fewer limitations due to heart failure as measured by the NYHA class, Minnesota Living with Heart Failure Questionnaire and clinical component of the Kansas City Cardiomyopathy Questionnaire. The incidences of several adverse events were lower as well including right heart failure, cardiac arrhythmias, device-related infections, sepsis, respiratory failure, renal failure and device replacement. None of the adverse events rates were higher in the HeartMate II group including major bleeding and strokes. This study provides moderate quality evidence that numerous patient outcomes in patients treated with the HeartMate II are better than the HeartMate XVE when used for destination therapy. Since patient characteristics and outcomes in the HeartMate XVE arm of this study were similar to those in the previous clinical trial that demonstrated the HeartMate XVE provided superior outcomes compared to optimal medical therapy,[2] one might infer that the HeartMate II would also be superior to optimal medical therapy.

A recent fair quality report[23] compared outcomes of patients enrolled in a continued access protocol to those who received the HeartMate II in the above randomized clinical trial (Appendix D, Table 1). Patient selection criteria and baseline characteristics in the continued access protocol were essentially the same as the randomized controlled trial. The patients enrolled in the continued access protocol had as good or better outcomes. After 24 months, the primary endpoint of survival free of disabling stroke or reoperation to remove the device was 50% in the group assigned to the HeartMate II in the randomized controlled trial versus 59% in the continued access protocol (p=0.07). Survival for 2 years was also similar 58% versus 63%, respectively. During follow-up survivors also had similar improvements in symptoms and related quality of life as measured by the NYHA class, Minnesota Living with Heart Failure Questionnaire and the Kansas City Cardiomyopathy Questionnaire. The incidences of hemorrhagic stroke, bleeding treated with packed red blood cells, sepsis and device-related infection were significantly lower in the group enrolled in the continued access protocol. The reduction in bleeding events was attributed to changes in the postoperative use of less aggressive anticoagulation regimens. There were no differences in the incidences of other adverse effects.

Two reports of case series[3,24] provided survival estimates for patients receiving the Heart Mate II as destination therapy (Appendix D, Table 1). Although these reports provided lower quality evidence, survival at one year in these cases series was similar to the 68% 1-year survival in the HeartMate II group in the randomized clinical trial. More recent survival estimates without heart transplantation or heart recovery from the INTERMACS registry that are based on 740 cases were 74% and approximately 60% after 1 and 2 years, respectively.[13] The available survival estimates are remarkably consistent with each other.

Summary of Findings for Key Question #1

A single good quality study provided evidence that use of the newer, continuous flow HeartMate II ventricular assist device for destination therapy provides better patient outcomes than the older, pulsatile flow HeartMate XVE device. A fair quality continued access protocol for use of the HeartMate II indicated that all of the reported patient outcomes continue to be as good as those seen in the randomized controlled trial or better including significantly fewer hemorrhagic strokes, major bleeding episodes and infections. Case series have also reported similar survival when the HeartMate II was used as destination therapy.

Clinical trials of other continuous flow devices for destination therapy such as a HeartWare device with a different continuous flow design are ongoing,[4,5,25] however results are not expected for several years.

KEY QUESTION #2. What patient or site characteristics have been associated with patient benefits or harms when the FDA-approved, current generation LVAD is used as destination therapy?

Based on the approved FDA indication and clinical trials, CMS has determined that the evidence is adequate to conclude that implantation of a left ventricular assist device approved by the FDA for destination therapy is reasonable and necessary for Medicare beneficiaries who have chronic end-stage heart failure, are not candidates for heart transplantation, and meet all of the following conditions: 1) NYHA Class IV symptoms of heart failure that have not responded to optimal medical management including dietary salt restriction, diuretics, digitalis, beta-blockers and angiotensin converting enzyme inhibitors (if not tolerated, presumably angiotensin receptor blockers would be an acceptable alternative) for at least 45 of the last 60 days or have been balloon pump dependent for 7 days, or IV inotrope dependent for 14 days (cardiac resynchronization therapy and an implantable cardiac defibrillator are not listed although they have become standards of care when clinically indicated for patients with heart failure), 2) a left ventricular ejection fraction less than 25%, 3) demonstrated functional limitation with a peak oxygen consumption of 14 ml/kg/min or less unless the patients is balloon pump or inotrope dependent or physically unable to perform an exercise test and 4) appropriate body size for the device.[12]

In addition, CMS determined that destination therapy is reasonable and necessary only when the procedure is performed in a facility approved under the Disease-Specific Care Certification Program for Ventricular Assist Device developed by the Joint Commission on Accreditation of Healthcare Organizations.[26] Facility staff must have implanted at least 10 ventricular assist devices or total artificial hearts as a bridge to transplant or as destination therapy during the past 36 months with at least one procedure within the past 18 months. The facility also must have in place staff and processes that assure that prospective recipients receive all information necessary to assist them in giving informed consent for the procedure, and so that they and their families are fully aware of the aftercare requirements and potential limitations as well as benefits. We found only one study of patient preferences related to use of ventricular assist devices that explored a few hypothetical situations describing life expectancy and daily function without the device.[27]

The CMS criteria also state that the facility must be an active, continuous member of a national, audited registry that requires submission of data on all destination therapy patients from the date of implantation throughout the remainder of the recipient's lives. The INTERMACS registry satisfies this CMS reporting requirement.

More detailed patient inclusion and exclusion criteria have been used in clinical trials of ventricular assist devices as destination therapy and are recommended by clinical experts.[28,29,30,31,32]

Since outcomes among patients meeting current selection criteria do vary, selection of patients could be refined using strong predictors of patient outcomes. Clearly, there is little or no benefit to patients that don't recover from the operation to implant a ventricular assist device. A validated method to determine which eligible patients have unacceptably high (not defined) operative risk might improve patient selection and outcomes. A report of INTERMACS data summarized in Appendix D, Table 2 indicated that the presence of cardiogenic shock, concomitant surgery and poorer renal function as indicated by higher blood urea nitrogen were associated with higher mortality within 30 days of the operation.[3] This analysis focused on use of ventricular devices as destination therapy but included many cases that received the obsolete HeartMate XVE. Interactions between the type of device and operative risk factors were not reported to determine whether the prognostic information depended on the type of device. More importantly, the risk factors were not used to identify patients that have an unacceptably high operative risk, and the confidence one would have in selecting patients based on the predicted probabilities of operative mortality risk was not reported.

Lietz et al. analyzed data in the manufacturer's registry of HeartMate XVE use post-FDA approval to develop a risk model of 90-day in hospital mortality.[11] The risk model incorporated several preoperative variables as summarized in Appendix D, Table 2. The risk score derived from this model discriminated the two outcome groups and could place patients into risk groups that had substantially different levels of risk. However, the difference in predicted and observed outcomes was substantial in some risk groups and the precision of the estimates was inadequate in the smaller risk groups. Furthermore, there was no consensus about which, if any, risk groups should be excluded from treatment due to high risk. We found no reports that tried to validate or update this risk model for current practices that use the HeartMate II device.

Current criteria for use of a ventricular assist device as destination therapy include an estimated 1-year survival without the device of less than 50%[14] or an overall life expectancy of less than 2 years.[10,12] A validated method for making these predictions has not been established. As summarized in Appendix D, Table 2, Levy et al. adapted and evaluated the Seattle Heart Failure Model to predict survival of the patients in the optimal medical therapy arm of the initial clinical trial of the HeartMate VE.[33] There was good agreement between the observed and predicted 1-year survival (28% versus 30%), and 81% met the guideline criterion of less than 50% predicted probability of survival for one year without a ventricular assist device. No further studies were found that indicated use of this prediction model would improve selection of patients for destination therapy or patient outcomes.

A secondary analysis of clinical trial data collected at a single center suggested that carefully selected patients that were 70 years old or older (a commonly used cutoff for heart transplantation) had similar outcomes to those less than 70 years old.[34] However as summarized in Appendix D, Table 2, there were only a small number of patients in this comparison and there were no adjustments for preoperative differences.

Summary of Findings for Key Question #2

The scientific evidence concerning use of newer generation, continuous flow FDA-approved ventricular assist devices, i.e., the HeartMate II, is insufficient to refine patient selection criteria for destination therapy beyond the current criteria used to enroll patients in the pivotal clinical trials and determine eligibility for CMS coverage.

A few studies have identified risk factors for mortality and developed or applied prediction models to this particular patient population. Further studies are needed to validate the use of different criteria to select patients and improve patient outcomes. An ongoing clinical trial is selecting less severely ill patients and may expand the criteria for use of a newer generation continuous flow devices as destination therapy.[4,5] In the meantime, the approved FDA indication and CMS criteria for coverage are available.

KEY QUESTION #3. What is the range of cost-effectiveness estimates of using the FDA-approved, current generation LVAD as destination therapy in end-stage heart failure and what explains variation in these estimates?

As reported in the results for Key Question #1, we identified one randomized trial comparing a current generation continuous flow ventricular assist device (HeartMate II) to the older generation (HeartMate XVE) ventricular assist device.[1] There was also one prior trial comparing an older generation HeartMate VE device to optimal medical management.[2] There have been no studies that directly compared a current generation device to optimal medical management. We found only one analysis of cost-effectiveness that used data from these two prior trials to indirectly estimate the cost-effectiveness of using the HeartMate II ventricular assist device for destination therapy compared to optimal medical management.[35]

Rogers et al. estimated that the continuous-flow device would have an incremental cost effectiveness ratio (ICER) of $198,184 per quality-adjusted life year and $167,208 per overall life years not adjusted for in the patients' quality of life.[35] Estimates of confidence intervals around these cost-effectiveness ratios were not reported. The analysis was funded by the maker of the device and the costs were assessed from the perspective of a third-party payer, not necessarily the VA. Details of this analysis related to the key model components, source data, and the effect sensitivity analyses are summarized in Appendix D, Table 3. The ICER estimates used "base case" assumptions regarding: survival that included the 24-month estimates from the clinical trials with extrapolation of survival thereafter, costs related to the initial implantation of the ventricular assist device, costs of medical management, re-hospitalization rates and costs, device replacement costs, outpatient care costs, end-of-life costs and estimates of quality of life (utility) for each of the four NYHA classes of limitations due to symptoms of heart failure that patients may fall in after implantation of the device. The quality of life assessment did not incorporate other medical conditions including the impact of device complications. Limited sensitivity analyses that changed one model component at a time suggested that the variation in the cost-effectiveness estimates were most dependent on the extrapolated estimates of survival from 24 to 60 months and the costs of the initial implantation of the ventricular assist device and subsequent re-hospitalizations for complications. Plausible changes to any of these individual assumptions resulted in estimates of cost-effectiveness ranging from $150,000 to $300,000 per quality-adjusted life year.

Prior analyses that compared use of the older generation ventricular assist device (HeartMate VE) to optimized medical management reported a cost-effectiveness ratio of $802,700 per quality-adjusted life year.[36] Rogers' adaptation of this model for the HeartMate II appeared to show a significant improvement in the cost-effectiveness. The main drivers of the improvement in cost-effectiveness were not well established, however, Rogers et al. state that the improvement was largely due to better survival, reductions in implant costs and better quality of life of surviving patients that received the device.[35] Nevertheless, destination therapy remains among the least cost-effective interventions covered by Medicare.[6]

Summary of Findings for Key Question #3

The estimated cost-effectiveness of using the HeartMate II as destination therapy for patients with end-stage heart failure was approximately $200,000 per quality-adjusted life year. The cost-effectiveness estimates did not drop below $150,000 even with more favorable assumptions regarding the outcomes or costs of using the HeartMate II ventricular assist device as destination therapy.

SUMMARY AND DISCUSSION

SUMMARY POINTS

- Only one good quality randomized trial of a newer generation continuous flow ventricular assist device as destination therapy has been reported to date. This study found that patients who received the HeartMate II had better survival, fewer major complications, spent less time in the hospital, and that their heart failure had substantially less adverse impact on their quality of life than those who received the older generation pulsatile flow HeartMate XVE device.

- Currently, selection of patients for destination therapy is based on the FDA approved indication and CMS criteria for coverage of Medicare beneficiaries that are based on enrollment criteria used by pivotal randomized controlled clinical trials. Studies have not validated use of other preoperative variables to further refine patient selection and thereby improve patient outcomes.

- Only one industry-funded cost-effectiveness analysis has been reported to date. This analysis reported costs from a third payer perspective and found that the incremental cost effective ratio was approximately $200,000 per quality-adjusted life year compared to optimal medical management.

LIMITATIONS

At this time there is limited, but encouraging, data to support use of the FDA approved continuous flow ventricular assist device as destination therapy. Only one randomized clinical trial has been completed. Patients enrolled in the clinical trial were carefully selected thereby limiting the ability to generalize the results. Outcomes continue to improve with experience in selecting patients, surgical procedures to implant ventricular assist devices and postoperative patient care.

The reviewed literature did not identify any VA medical center that has enrolled patients in a clinical trial or the national INTERMACS registry. The number of veterans who would meet the current selection criteria for using a left ventricular assist device as destination therapy is not known. Additional data and analyses are needed to estimate the costs the Veterans Health Administration would incur to provide this highly-specialized care.

RECOMMENDATIONS FOR FUTURE RESEARCH

Additional high-quality data are needed to inform clinical practices and policies regarding the use of ventricular assist devices to treat patients with end-stage heart failure who are not eligible for a heart transplant. Investigators suggest the following recommendations regarding future research:

- **Create or participate in a registry of all Veterans that receive an LVAD as destination therapy, and support enrollment of Veterans in ongoing, randomized controlled clinical trials.**

    Given the small number of patients who have received destination therapy and the rapidly evolving devices and practices, it is imperative to learn as much as possible from patients who undergo this procedure. All Veterans that receive destination therapy approved by the Veterans Health Administration should be entered into a national registry in a way that will allow separate analyses and comparisons of patient characteristics and outcomes. In addition, enrollment of patients into randomized controlled clinical trials should be encouraged. For example, a study comparing a third generation ventricular assist device to FDA-approved devices is currently trying to enroll up to 450 patients who, for the most part, meet current criteria for destination therapy.[25] As ventricular assist devices become more durable with fewer complications they are also being tested in patients with less severe heart failure given concerns that the operative risk of many patients who meet the current criteria for destination therapy is too high, and patients with a less dire prognosis without a device may benefit from increasingly reliable devices.[4,5] Permission to enroll patients in this study of a currently unapproved use of a newer device (HeartWare) should be considered to increase patient access to destination therapy.

- **Validate and, if necessary, update prediction models especially for early post-operative mortality.**

  Patients who die in the hospital soon after implantation of a ventricular assist device do not benefit. A validated prediction model for early/postoperative mortality could be applied to avoid high risk and costly attempts to use ventricular assist devices as destination therapy. Ideally clinical trials would be done to show that use of an outcome prediction model improves patient outcomes. This review did not find any established or proposed threshold for predicted risk of post operative mortality that would preclude use of destination therapy or generally be acceptable to patients and health care providers.

- **Develop decision aids to help providers share information about the benefits, risks and care needed when using an approved ventriclualr assist device as destination therapy and to help them make decisions that are consistent with the informed patient's values and preferences.**

  The difficult decision to employ a ventricular assist device as destination therapy typically is made when patients are in poor health and have a very limited life expectancy without the device. A number of benefits and risks need to be explained in ways patients can understand including the uncertainty inherent in the outcomes data. Patients need to understand the follow-up care that will be required. Future states of health when the patient might want the device to be turned off need to be anticipated and discussed. Decisions aids can enhance provider-patient communication and increase patients' knowledge and participation and acceptance of the decision.[37]

- **Update the cost-effectiveness model as more data become available and incorporate a probabilistic sensitivity analysis.**

  There have been large improvements in the cost-effectiveness of destination therapy during the past decade.[35,36] It will be important to keep updating the cost-effectiveness models as the devices and related procedures improve. This is particularly important for the model parameters that appear to be most influential i.e., long-term survival both on the device and with optimal medical management, cost of the device, cost of initial hospitalization, rehospitalization rate and utility estimates based on measures of health-related quality of life. Additionally, adding probabilistic sensitivity modeling would help decision makers better understand the uncertainty of the estimates in the model by estimating confidence intervals around the incremental cost-effectiveness estimates. This can be done by using distributions of the model parameters with Monte Carlo simulation to assess the probability the incremental cost effectieness ratio will be less than or greater than various dollar amounts. Probabilistic sensitivity analyses that took the UK National Health Service payer perspective have been completed for the cost-effectiveness of continous flow LVAD as a bridge to transplant providing a good example of what could be done for destination therapy.[38]

- **Conduct a budget impact analysis.**

    Cost-effectiveness analyses provide general estimates from a societal perspective or the perspective of a generic third party payer, however, additional budget impact analyses would be useful to help the Veterans Health Administration understand the potential impact of different strategies and policies for providing destination therapy. For example, it would be important to know how many veterans would be eligible and interested in the treatment and what the options would be in terms of how and where this therapy would be provided.

CONCLUSIONS

Key Question #1
Use of the FDA-approved HeartMate II rather than the HeartMate XVE left ventricular assist device results in superior patient outcomes (better survival and daily existence, fewer harmful complications). [moderate strength evidence]

Key Question #2
Preoperative correlates of patient outcomes have not been established as patient selection criteria that can lead to better patient outcomes. [insufficient evidence]

Key Question #3
The cost-effectiveness of HeartMate II ventricular assist device for destination therapy has been estimated to be approximately $200,000 per quality-adjusted life year when compared to optimal medical management. [low strength evidence]

REFERENCES

1. Slaughter MS, Rogers JG, Milano CA, et al. for the HeartMate II Investigators. Advanced heart failure treated with continuous-flow left ventricular assist devices. *N Engl J Med.* 2009;361:2241-51.

2. Rose EA, Gellins AC, Moskowitz AJ, et al. for the REMATCH Study Group. Long-term use of a left ventricular assist device for end-stage heart failure. *N Engl J Med.* 2001;345:1435-43.

3. Kirklin JK, Naftel DC, Kormos RL, et al. Third INTERMACS annual report: The evolution of destination therapy in the United States. *J Heart Lung Transplant.* 2011;30:115-23.

4. Baldwin JT, Mann DL. NHLBI's program for VAD therapy for moderately advanced heart failure: The REVIVE-IT pilot trial. *J Card Fail.* 2010;16:855-8.

5. ClinicalTrials.gov. The evaluation of VAD InterVEntion before inotropic therapy (REVIVE-IT). NCT01369407. Available at http://clinicaltrials.gov/ct2/show/record/NCT01369407. Accessed December 19, 2011.

6. Chambers JD, Neumann PJ, Buxton MJ. Does Medicare have an implicit cost-effectiveness threshold? *Med Decis Making.* 2010;30(4):E14-E27.

7. Miller LW. Is left ventricular assist device therapy underutilized in the treatment of heart failure? *Circulation.* 2011;123:1552-8.

8. Terracciano CM, Miller LW, Yacoub MH. Contemporary use of ventricular assist devices. *Annu Rev Med.* 2010;61:255-70.

9. John R, Naka Y, Smedira NG, et al. Continuous flow left ventricular assist device outcomes in commercial use compared with the prior clinical trial. *Ann Thorac Surg.* 2011;92:1406-13.

10. FDA Device Approvals and Clearances. HeartMate® SNAP-VE LVAS - P920014/S016. Available at http://www.accessdata.fda.gov/cdrh_docs/pdf/p920014s016a.pdf. Accessed April 27, 2012.

11. Lietz K, Long JW, Kfoury AG, et al. Outcomes of left ventricular assist device implantation as destination therapy in the post-REMATCH era. *Circulation.* 2007;116:497-505.

12. Centers for Medicare & Medicaid Services. Decision Memo for Ventricular Assist Devices as Destination Therapy (CAG-00119N) issued in October 2003 with revisions in March 2007 (CAG-00119R1) and November 2010 (CAG-00119R2). Available at https://www.cms.gov/medicare-coverage-database/details/nca-decision-memo.aspx?NCAId=79&ver=6&NcaName=Ventricular+Assist+Devices+as+Destination+Therapy&bc=BEAAAAAAEAAA&&fromdb=true. Accessed December 2, 2011.

13. Kirklin JK, Naftel DC, Kormos RL, et al. Fourth INTERMACS annual report: 4,000 implants and counting. *J Heart Lung Transplant.* 2012;31:117-26.

14. Jessup M, Abraham WT, Casey DE, et al. writing on behalf of the 2005 Guideline Update for the Diagnosis and Management of Chronic Heart Failure in the Adult Writing Committee. 2009 Focused update: ACCF/AHA guidelines for the diagnosis and management of heart failure in adults. *Circulation.* 2009;119:1977-2016.

15. Lindenfeld J, Albert NM, Boehmer JP, et al. HFSA 2010 Comprehensive Heart Failure Practice Guideline. Available at http://www.heartfailureguideline.org. Accessed December 2, 2011.

16. McKelvie RS, Moe GW, Cheung A, et al. The 2011 Canadian Cardiovascular Society heart failure management guidelines updates: Focus on sleep apnea, renal dysfunction, mechanical circulatory support, and palliative care. *Can J Cardiol.* 2011;27:319-38.

17. Parides MK, Moskowitz AJ, Ascheim DD, Rose EA, Gelijns AC. Progress versus precision: Challenges in clinical trial design for left ventricular assist devices. *Ann Thorac Surg.* 2006;82:1140-6.

18. Patel-Raman SM, Chen EA. Past, present, and future regulatory aspects of ventricular assist devices. *J Cardiovasc Transl Res.* 2010;3:600-3.

19. Neaton JD, Normand S-L, Gelijns A, Starling RC, Mann DL, Konstam MA. Designs for mechanical circulatory support device studies. *J Cardiac Fail.* 2007;13:63-74.

20. Higgins JPT, Green S, eds. Cochrane Handbook for Systematic Reviews of Interventions Version 5.1.0 (updated March 2011): The Cochrane Collaboration; 2011: Available at http://www.cochrane-handbook.org/. Accessed August 29, 2011.

21. Sculpher M, Fenwick E, Claxton K. Assessing quality in decision analytic cost-effectiveness models. A suggested framework and example of application. *Pharmacoeconomics.* 2000;17:461-77.

22. Owens DK, Lohr KN, Atkins D, et al. AHRQ series paper 5: grading the strength of a body of evidence when comparing medical interventions--agency for healthcare research and quality and the effective health-care program. *J Clin Epidemiol.* 2010;63(5):513-523.

23. Park SJ, Milano CA, Tatooles AJ, et al. for the HeartMate II Clinical Investigators. Outcomes in advanced heart failure patients with left ventricular assist devices for destination therapy. *Circ Heart Fail.* 2012 Jan 26;Epub ahead of print.

24. Strüber M, Kander K, Lahpor J, et al. HeartMate II left ventricular assist device; early European experience. *Eur J Cardiothorac Surg.* 2008;34:289-94.

25. ClinicalTrials.gov. A clinical trial to evaluate the HeartWare® ventricular assist system (ENDURANCE). NCT01166347. Available at http://clinicaltrials.gov/ct2/show/record/NCT01166347. Accessed December 8, 2011.

26. Joint Commission, The. Advanced Certification in Ventricular Assist Device. Available at http://www.jointcommission.org/certification/ventricular_assist_device.aspx. Accessed March 2, 2012.

27. Stewart CG, Brooks K, Pratibhu PP, et al. Thresholds of physical activity and life expectancy for patients considering destination ventricular assist devices. *J Heart Lung Transplant.* 2009;28:863-9.

28. Lietz K, Miller LW. Patient selection for left-ventricular assist devices. *Curr Opin Cardiol.* 2009;24:246-51.

29. Lietz K. Destination therapy: patient selection and current outcomes. *J Card Surg.* 2010;25:462-71.

30. Slaughter MS, Pagani FD, Rogers JG, et al. for the HeartMate II Clinical Investigators. Clinical management of continuous-flow left ventricular assist devices in advanced heart failure. *J Heart Lung Transplant.* 2010;29:S1-S39.

31. Tang DG, Oyer PE, Mallidi HR. Ventricular assist devices: History, patient selection, and timing of therapy. *J Cardiovasc Transl Res.* 2009;2:159-67.

32. Wilson SR, Mudge GH, Stewart GC, Givertz MM. Evaluation for a ventricular assist device. *Circulation.* 2009;119:2225-32.

33. Levy WC, Mozaffarian D, Linker DT, Farrar DJ, Miller LW, on behalf of the REMATCH Investigators. Can the Seattle Heart Failure Model be used to risk-stratify heart failure patients for potential left ventricular assist device therapy? *J Heart Lung Transplant.* 2009;28:231-6.

34. Adamson RM, Stahovich M, Chillcott S, et al. Clinical strategies and outcomes in advanced heart failure patients older than 70 years of age receiving the HeartMate II left ventricular assist device. *J Am Coll Cardiol.* 2011;57:2487-95.

35. Rogers JG, Bostic RR, Tong KB, Adamson R, Russo M, Slaughter MS. Cost-effectiveness analysis of continuous-flow left ventricular assist devices as destination therapy. *Circulation:Heart Fail.* 2012;5:10-6.

36. Samson D. Special report: cost-effectiveness of left-ventricular assist devices as destination therapy for end-stage heart failure. *Technology Evaluation Center Assessment Program Report.* 2004;19:1-36.

37. Allen LA, Stevenson LW, Grady KL, et al. Decision making in advanced heart failure, a scientific statement from the American Heart Association. *Circulation.* 2012;125:00-00 online ahead of print DOI: 10.1161/CIR.0b013e31824f2173.

38. Moreno SG, Novielli N, Cooper NJ. Cost-effectiveness of the implantable HeartMate II left ventricular assist device for patients awaiting heart transplantation. *J Heart Lung Transplant.* 2012:31(5):450-8.

APPENDIX A. TECHNICAL EXPERT PANEL MEMBERS

Inder Anand, MD, FRCP, DPhil
Director, Heart Failure Program
University of Minnesota Medical School

William Gunnar, MD, JD
National Director of Surgery
Department of Veterans Affairs

William Holman, MD
Chief, Surgical Services
Birmingham VA Medical Center

Gundars Katlaps, MD
Chief, Section of Cardiothoracic Surgery
Surgical Director, Programs of Heart Transplantation and Mechanical Assist Devices
Richmond McGuire VA Medical Center

Richard Schofield, MD, FACC
Chairman of Medicine
Malcolm Randal VA Medical Center
Chief, Medical Service
North Florida/South Georgia Veterans Health System

Josef Stehlik, MD
Director, VAMC Cardiac Transplant Program
VA Salt Lake City Health Care System

APPENDIX B. SEARCH STRATEGY

Database: Ovid MEDLINE(R) <1948 to October Week 3 2011>

Search Strategy:

----

1   exp Heart-Assist Devices/ or lvad.mp.
2   ventric$ assist.mp.
3   artificial ventricle.mp.
4   heartware.mp.
5   heartmate.mp.
6   novacor.mp.
7   coraide.mp.
8   lionheart.mp.
9   or/1-8
10   limit 9 to (english language and humans and yr="1995 -Current")
11   congestive heart failure.mp. or exp Heart Failure/ or cardiac failure.mp. or myocardial failure.mp. or ventricular dysfunction.mp. or exp Ventricular Dysfunction/
12   10 and 11
13   limit 12 to (case reports or comment or editorial or letter)
14   12 not 13

APPENDIX C. PEER REVIEW COMMENTS/AUTHOR RESPONSES

REVIEWER COMMENT	RESPONSE
1. Are the objectives, scope, and methods for this review clearly described?	
Yes. This is a very well written report that reviewing the evidence available for the use of the current generation of left ventricular assist devices as destination therapy. Given the very limited published data on the subject, the authors have adequately addressed the three key questions required for this topic.	
Yes	
Yes	
Yes. The methods are clearly described and are standard for this type of evaluation. However, it should be noted that there are factors inherent in ventricular assist devices (VADs) that importantly influence their evaluation in clinical trials. First, the control group in trials to date (e.g. optimal medical management group of the REMATCH trial) is critically ill. Survival of the control group in REMATCH was so poor that a medical control group will be considered ethically unacceptable for subsequent trials, unless the trial specifically examines less ill patients (e.g. the The Evaluation of VAD InterVEntion Before Inotropic Therapy [REVIVE-IT] trial cited in the report, which will examine class IIIB patients). The REVIVE-IT trial itself faces challenges with regard to patients that cross-over from medical to device management during the trial. Clinical trials of new VADs for class IV heart failure will use approved devices as the control group. The report recognizes this situation and its limitations. A second factor stems from the fact that the therapy cannot be blinded to the observers or the patient. The use of objective measures such as maximal oxygen consumption and six minute walk test is therefore particularly important to trials and their evaluation	We have added a statement about use of more objective endpoints to the section on page 11 about patient outcomes for KQ1. We believe that although more objective endpoints such as exercise tests would be useful given the inability to blind comparisons between devices and non-surgical medical therapy, it is very difficult to translate changes in maximal exercise test parameters to effects on patients' lives. Subjective patient outcomes could be less of an issue in unblinded comparisons of devices.
Yes	
Yes. I found this review to be well-written and focused. The objectives of the review were clearly defined, and were presented in logical and concise manner. The scope of the review was also well described and took proper account for lack of sufficient data to definitively answer one of the key points. The methods applied to the project were reasonable and consistent with evidence-based analysis of the data.	
Yes. Objectives, scope and methods are clearly described and appropriate for the potential therapy being evaluated.	
2. Is there any indication of bias in our synthesis of the evidence?	
No	
No	
No	
No	
No	
No. I could not perceive a detectable bias in the synthesis of the evidence. The authors are to be commended for a balanced approach to the key questions posed	
No. Evaluation appears to be free of any bias and the Technical Expert Panel Members are noted experts capable of providing appropriate guidance and oversight	

Use of Left Ventricular Assist Devices as Destination Therapy
in End-Stage Congestive Heart Failure: A Systematic Review

REVIEWER COMMENT	RESPONSE
3. Are there any published or unpublished studies that we may have overlooked?	
Yes. The authors have reviewed most of the published and unpublished data on the subject from 1995 to October 2011. However, it would be useful to include in this document the additional information in the latest Quarterly Statistical Report from the Interagency Registry for Mechanically Assisted Circulatory Support (INTERMACS) available on their web site. According to this report, the total number of medical centers performing LVAD implantations for destination therapy have doubled from 69 to 135 as quoted by the authors (page 7, para 3, line 6). Moreover, over a fifth of all LVADs have been implanted for destination therapy.	Updated information from the fourth annual INTERMACS report has been added to the Registry section on page 7. In addition, the INTERMACS website is now referenced there to provide access to up-to-date information.
No. There are limited publications related to HeartMate II	
No	
Yes. The fourth INTERMACS report was published in the February issue of the Journal of Heart and Lung Transplantation. The information will not dramatically change the findings of the VA-ESP report, in my opinion. However, the report may want to include the citation.	Updated information from the fourth annual INTERMACS report has been added to the Registry section on page 7. In addition, the INTERMACS website is now referenced there to provide access to up to date information.
The HeartWare left ventricular assist device is currently under review by the FDA for the bridge-to-transplantation indication. It may be worth mentioning this device as a future consideration, primarily due to the pump's small size. It was chosen for the REVIVE-IT trial.	We have now mentioned the HeartWare by name when discussing ongoing studies on pages 3, 17 and 23.
Yes 1) Ann Thorac Surg. 2011 Nov;92(5):1593-9; discussion 1599-600. Epub 2011 Oct 31. **Lessons learned from experience with over 100 consecutive HeartMate II left ventricular assist devices.** John R, Kamdar F, Eckman P, Colvin-Adams M, Boyle A, Shumway S, Joyce L, Liao K.	The first report listed was screened but not included in this review because only 17 out of the 130 cases were destination therapy.
2) J Heart Lung Transplant. 2011 Aug;30(8):849-53. Epub 2011 Apr 29. **Arteriovenous malformation and gastrointestinal bleeding in patients with the HeartMate II left ventricular assist device.** Demirozu ZT, Radovancevic R, Hochman LF, Gregoric ID, Letsou GV, Kar B, Bogaev RC, Frazier OH.	The second report listed was screened but not included in this review because most cases were not destination therapy. The article does point out the need to consider the risk and incidence of gastrointestinal bleeding as an important patient outcome particularly with continuous flow devices. Information about this important patient outcome was extracted whenever it was reported by studies that were included in the review.
3) J Heart Lung Transplant. 2012 Jan;31(1):1-8. Epub 2011 Oct 8. **Pre-operative and post-operative risk factors associated with neurologic complications in patients with advanced heart failure supported by a left ventricular assist device.** Kato TS, Schulze PC, Yang J, Chan E, Shahzad K, Takayama H, Uriel N, Jorde U, Farr M, Naka Y, Mancini D.	The third report listed was published after the literature search was done. It was not included this review because most cases used the older pulsatile flow HeartMate device that has become obsolete. Furthermore, the report doesn't provide enough information to determine the predictive accuracy of identified risk factors for neurological complications. Judging by the magnitude of the differences, most likely the identified risk factors will not turn out to provide adequate discrimination. The article does point out the need to consider the risk and incidence of neurological complications as an important patient outcome. Information about this important patient outcome was extracted whenever it was reported by studies that were included in the review.
4) Ann Thorac Surg. 2010 Oct;90(4):1270-7. **Infectious complications in patients with left ventricular assist device: etiology and outcomes in the continuous-flow era.** Topkara VK, Kondareddy S, Malik F, Wang IW, Mann DL, Ewald GA, Moazami N.	The fourth report listed was screened but not included this review because most cases weren't destination therapy, and the report doesn't provide much information about patient selection based on the risk of infectious complications. The article does point out the need to consider the risk and incidence of infectious complications as an important patient outcome. Information about this important patient outcome was extracted whenever it was reported by studies that were included in the review.

Use of Left Ventricular Assist Devices as Destination Therapy in End-Stage Congestive Heart Failure: A Systematic Review

Evidence-based Synthesis Program

REVIEWER COMMENT	RESPONSE
Yes. The authors may wish to review the following citation: "Moreno SG, Novielli N, Cooper NJ. Cost-effectiveness of the implantable left ventricular assist device HeartMate II for patients awaiting heart transplantation. J Heart Lung Transplant March 2012 (e-published ahead of print)", and the accompanying editorial by MS Slaughter and JG Rogers, titled "Determining the cost-effectiveness of mechanical circulatory support"	We have carefully reviewed both of these citations and decided against adding this cost-effectiveness analysis to the results section of the report because it took a UK National Health Service payer perspective and only looked at LVAD use as a bridge to heart transplant, However, the Moreno 2012 article does provide a good example of what could be done in a future in terms of a probabilistic cost-effectiveness analysis, so we incorporated information about this study into the Recommendations for Future Research Section on page 24.
No. There are no significant publications that have been overlooked or additional publications not included that would add value to the evaluation of in any way change the conclusions that have been made.	
4. Additional suggestions or comments	
Minor comments: Page 4 bullet # 3, line3; correct "ventricular" Page 35, column 4; it is unclear for which comparison the HR for all –cause death within 30 days refers to? Page 37, column 4; Mean pulmonary pressure > or ≤ 25 mmHg?	Typographical error on page 4 corrected. The reference groups for the HR's now have been noted. The article repeatedly states ≤ 25 as indicated. The authors considered a low mean pulmonary artery pressure to be an indicator of right heart failure although others have associated worse outcomes with higher pulmonary pressures that can precipitate right heart failure after implantation of a left ventricular assist device.
On page 23 you state "A consensus of health care providers and patients needs to be established for the level of predicted mortality that would generally preclude use of destination therapy." Ideally, this would be based on data from randomized trials directly. Estimating the risk benefit of a VAD on sub-populations without trial data has a high potential for error. If economic studies determine a minimum survival threshold that must be achieved in order for VAD implantation to be cost-effective then it would be useful to develop studies to predict survival less than that threshold.	We agree and have revised the statement on page 23 to, "Ideally clinical trials would be done to show that use of a prediction model improves patient outcomes. This review did not find any established or proposed threshold for predicted risk that would preclude use of destination therapy or generally be acceptable to patients and health care providers."
For your recommendation to register patients I would state the name/details of registry as many will not read the text to figure out what you are talking about. They may assume you are suggesting the VA could/ should start its own registry.	The INTERMACS registry has now been specified.
The report was well written with appropriate supporting literature. With regard to Key Question #2, information from INTERMACS defines risk factors for death following implantation of a ventricular assist device. At this point in time, the information has not been reduced to a quantitative predictive nomogram, but probably will be in the near future. Dr. David Naftel at UAB can give the group a better estimation of the timeline for developing a system to predict outcome in mechanical circulatory assist patients. I have no additional comments or suggestions	

Use of Left Ventricular Assist Devices as Destination Therapy in End-Stage Congestive Heart Failure: A Systematic Review

REVIEWER COMMENT	RESPONSE
I've added several references describing outcomes AFTER the clinical studies were concluded. You can see that outcomes are not as good for patients getting devices WITHOUT being enrolled in clinical studies. This is not an observation unique to this particular clinical problem, but I think it warrants more attention.	Points well taken. Observational studies that directly compared outcomes in practice versus clinical trials were of interest as were reports of patient outcomes in case series. Many of these reports were from investigational sites and we couldn't always tell if the report included or excluded patients that were enrolled in clinical trials. Hopefully, the INTERMACS registry data will provide better estimates of the incidences of all types of patient outcomes. The articles did not identify any additional patient outcomes that were not considered during the review.
I noticed that the comparison focused on the comparison of newer devices to older ones, based on the assumption that LVAD's generally have been shown to improve survival v. nonsurgical management. But what about other outcomes? There is an alarming incidence of disabling strokes in patients with LVAD's. How would this figure in a patient's decision to have an LVAD implanted? Would patient's be willing to accept a higher mortality with nonsurgical management in order to avoid the increased likelihood of a disabling stroke if an LVAD is implanted? (For this reason, issues of informed consent also warrant attention. Are patients being made aware of the high complication rates before agreeing to implantation? (I appreciate this was not part of the charge of the committee.)	
Regarding Key Question 1, there is no debate that use of the HeartMate II LVAD as compared to the HeartMate XVE LVAD in appropriate candidates leads to better outcomes, and that if compared to medical therapy alone the outcomes would be more decidedly favorable. However it would be important for the reviewers to point out that overall survival for DT patients with a HeartMate II was still only 55% at 2 years. This point would be of relevance to readers of the review and to policy makers. It is possible, perhaps even likely, that subsequent registry data will show improvement in the 2 year survival for DT patients supported via HeartMate II devices. If future updates to this report are generated, such data would be of considerable importance and should be disseminated. I am aware of anecdotes reporting very high 1 year survival rates for DT LVAD patients (I believe from the INTERMACS data set) but to my knowledge these data are not yet published.	The outcomes of using the HeartMate II as destination therapy study including the overall survival are summarized in the Executive Summary (page 3) and in the body of the report and evidence table. We have also cited other survival estimates in the report and added updated 2-year estimates from the INTERMACS registry on page 17. All estimates appear to be remarkably consistent with a trend to improved survival as patient selection and processes improve.
Are there data regarding readmission rates for patients who have undergone DT LVAD implantation? Such data would also be of interest to VA leadership. High rates of readmission post-operatively could mitigate some of the otherwise considerable advantages of LVAD placement in this very ill population of patients. I am aware of anecdotal reports that LVAD patients average >5 hospital readmissions over the first postoperative year, but these are purely anecdotes. Data in this regard might be useful.	Our search did not find good estimates of readmission rates or what complications caused them. The cost effectiveness estimates do include readmission rates of 0.21 per month for device therapy versus 0.13 for medical therapy, and the cost effectiveness ratio was sensitive to the presumed readmission rate as has been pointed out in the report.
I would agree with the authors that any patient who receives a DT LVAD via the Veterans Administration should be put into a robust data registry and that patient outcomes should be followed over time. I would submit that these patients perhaps should be entered into the VA surgical quality improvement database, which is strong and robust and already is established at every VA hospital with a surgical program on site. I would also consider whether current LVADs being placed by the VA as bridge to transplant should also be entered into a clinical database in order to track outcomes.	The VA surgical quality improvement data base has been added to the recommendation.
On page 7, paragraph 1 of the report, the authors note criteria established by the Centers for Medicare and Medicaid Services for clinical centers planning to initiate a DT LVAD program. The criteria included participation in a data registry, minimum volume standards for the implanting surgeon, and facility disease-specific certification for VADs by The Joint Commission. While VA would probably not be compelled to follow such CMS guidelines, one wonders whether it would nevertheless be wise and prudent to do so both to insure quality of the program and to deflect external criticism which might be directed at the VA for undertaking such a complex endeavor.	We agree, and had summarized the CMS criteria and other guidelines in the report to facilitate consideration by VA policymakers.

Use of Left Ventricular Assist Devices as Destination Therapy in End-Stage Congestive Heart Failure: A Systematic Review

Evidence-based Synthesis Program

REVIEWER COMMENT	RESPONSE
My only additional comment would pertain to Key Question #2 regarding site characteristics associated with patient benefits or harm. There is a trend in the U.S for "non-transplant" centers to establish stand-alone LVAD DT programs. It is unclear if these programs that have minimal to no transplant experience and have little to no experience with implanting LVADs as BTT will have similar outcomes in an older and potentially sicker DT patient population. It is possible that the VA system will need to address the question of whether it is feasible, makes clinical or economic sense to allow a LVAD DT program in a VA hospital without an advanced heart failure program that includes experience and expertise in the evaluation of heart transplant patients. Hopefully there will be some data in the next 3 – 5 years to help resolve this issue.	
5. Please provide any recommendations on how this report can be revised to more directly address or assist implementation needs.	
Provide emphasis regarding how remarkable technologic advancements have resulted in improved device outcomes. CMS did not consider conditional reimbursement until after the Slaughter study was published.	
No changes are needed.	
I think that the report accurately depicts the status quo of mechanical circulatory support.	
The Joint Commission has a process for accrediting mechanical circulatory support programs that may be of interest to the Veterans Administration. The requirements for this specialized accreditation describe in detail the personnel, processes, and infra-structure that are required for a mechanical circulatory support program	
The authors are to be congratulated for creation of a balanced, thoughtful and well written report.	
No additional recommendations	

APPENDIX D. EVIDENCE TABLES

Table 1. Key Question #1: Effects on Patient Outcomes

Study/Country/ Funding Source	Inclusion/Exclusion Criteria	Baseline Characteristics	Comparison	Patient Outcomes	Study Quality
Slaughter 2009[1] 38 centers in U.S. Funding Source: Manufacturer Thoratec	Inclusion Criteria: Ineligible for heart transplant Refractory to optimal medical care Left ventricular ejection fraction <25% Peak oxygen consumption <14ml/kg/min if able to exercise NYHA class IIIb or IV symptoms for 45 out of last 60 days, or IABP for 7 days, or intravenous inotrope for 14 days Exclusion Criteria: Inordinately high surgical risk Body mass index > 40 kg/m² Previous heart transplant Psychiatric condition or otherwise impaired protocol compliance Severe respiratory disease Serum creatinine ≥ 3.5 mg% or chronic dialysis Any other condition that could limit survival to < 3 years Several others not listed here	n = 200 Mean Age (yr): 62 Male: 84% White: 74% Mean LVEF: 17% IV inotrope: 79% IABP: 22% Mech. Vent.: 8% ICD: 82% CRT: 60% NYHA class: III - 22% IV - 69%	Investigational (I): HeartMate II continuous flow LVAD with warfarin (n=134) (1 received the control LVAD) Control (C): HeartMate XVE pulsatile flow LVAD without warfarin (n=66) (3 received the investigational LVAD) Median time on LVAD: I – 1.7 years C – 0.6 years	Primary composite endpoint of survival free of disabling stroke or reoperation to remove device including urgent heart transplant at 24 months I – 46% vs C – 11% (p<0.001) HR = 0.38 (95% CI 0.27 to 0.54) First events: Death I - 33% vs C – 41% (p=0.05) HR = 0.59 (95% CI 0.35 to 0.99) Device Removed I - 10% vs C – 36% (p<0.001) HR = 0.18 (95% CI 0.09 to 0.37) Disabling Stroke I - 11% vs C – 12% (p=0.56) HR = 0.78 (95% CI 0.33 to .82) As treated actuarial 1 and 2 year survival estimates ignoring device replacements (overall p=0.008 with HR = 0.54 (95% CI 0.34 to 0.86)) I (n=133): 68% (1 year) and 58% (2 year) C (n=59): 55% (1 year) and 24% (2 year) % of follow-up time spent as outpatient I – 88% vs C – 74% (p=0.02) Median initial length of stay I – 27 vs C – 28 days Readmission rate (per person year) I – 2.6 vs C – 4.2 (p=0.02)	Randomized Groups similar at baseline with no need for further adjustment Not blinded Withdrawals explained Intention to Treat (ITT) analysis of primary outcome; other outcomes analyzed as treated Adequate number and precision of estimates

Use of Left Ventricular Assist Devices as Destination Therapy in End-Stage Congestive Heart Failure: A Systematic Review

Study/Country/ Funding Source	Inclusion/Exclusion Criteria	Baseline Characteristics	Comparison	Patient Outcomes	Study Quality

Slaughter 2009[1] Continued	See above	See above	See above	<u>NYHA class I/II among survivors at 1-year</u>
				I (n=72) - 76% vs C (n=18) - 61%) (p=0.22)
				
				<u>Mean LHFQ Score among survivors at 1-year (lower better)</u>
				I (n=76) - 34 vs C (n=19) - 44 (p=0.03)
				
				<u>Mean KCCQ Clinical Score among survivors at 1-year (higher better)</u>
				I (n=76) - 69 vs C (n=18) - 61 (p=0.12)
				
				<u>Selected Adverse Event Rates (per person yr)</u>
				                      I C p-value
				Stroke 0.1 0.5 <0.001
				Sepsis 0.4 1.1 <0.001
				Major bleed 1.6 2.4 0.06
				Right heart failure
				                     0.1 0.5 <0.001
				Respiratory failure
				                     0.3 0.8 <0.001
				Cardiac arrhythmia requiring treatment
				                     0.7 1.3 0.006
				Renal failure 0.1 0.3 <0.001
					See above

Use of Left Ventricular Assist Devices as Destination Therapy in End-Stage Congestive Heart Failure: A Systematic Review

Study/Country/ Funding Source	Inclusion/Exclusion Criteria	Baseline Characteristics	Comparison	Patient Outcomes	Study Quality

Park 2012[23]
 	
38 centers in U.S.
 	
Funding Source: Manufacturer Thoratec
	Continued access protocol with same inclusion/exclusion criteria as previous study (Slaughter 2009[1])	n = 414
		Mean Age (yr): 63
		Male: 79%
		Mean LVEF: 17%
		IV inotrope: 78%
		IABP: 20%
		Mech. Vent.: 5%
		ICD: 83%
		CRT: 61%
		NYHA class:
		III – 34%
		IV – 66%
		
		Predicted 1-year survival without device: 41%
			All received HeartMate II
			
			Early enrollees (EE) in RCT from 3/2005 to 5/2007 (n=133), reported previously
			
			Later enrollees (LE) in non-randomized continued access protocol from 5/2007 to 3/2009 (n=281)
			
			Median duration of device use:
			EE 1.7 vs LE 2.1 yrs
				Primary composite endpoint - survival free of disabling stroke or reoperation to remove device including urgent heart transplant at 24 months
				EE – 50% vs LE – 59% (p=0.07)
				
				Actuarial 1 and 2 year survival
				EE: 68% (1 year) and 58% (2 year)
				LE: 73% (1 year) and 63% (2 year)
				overall p=0.21
				
				Median initial length of stay
				EE – 27 vs LE – 23 days (p=0.09)
				
				Readmission rate (per person year)
				I – 2.6 vs C – 4.2 (p=0.02)
				
				NYHA class I or II among survivors at 1-year
				EE (n=73) - 77% vs LE (n=161) - 77%
				
				Mean LHFQ Score among survivors at 6-months (lower better)
				EE (n=86) - 30 vs LE (n=184) - 38 over 2 years p=0.04
				
				Mean overall KCCQ Score among survivors at 6-months (higher better)
				EE (n=86) - 64 vs LE (n=187) - 70 over 2 years p=0.08
				
				Selected Adverse Event Rates (per person yr)
				                             EE LE p-value
				Ischemic stroke 0.06 0.05 0.48
				Hemorr. stroke 0.07 0.03 0.01
				Sepsis 0.38 0.27 0.02
				Device infection 0.47 0.27 <0.001
				Major bleed 1.89 1.27 <0.01
				Right heart failure 0.16 0.13 0.39
				Cardiac arrhythmia requiring treatment
				                              0.69 0.46 <0.01
				Renal failure 0.10 0.06 0.11
				Pump replacement 0.06 0.04 0.35
					Not randomized
					Groups similar at baseline with no need for further adjustment
					Not blinded
					Withdrawals not explained
					Intention to Treat (ITT) analysis
					Adequate number and precision of estimates

Use of Left Ventricular Assist Devices as Destination Therapy in End-Stage Congestive Heart Failure: A Systematic Review

Study/Country/ Funding Source	Inclusion/Exclusion Criteria	Baseline Characteristics	Comparison	Patient Outcomes	Study Quality
Kirklin 2011[3] 3rd INTERMACS Annual Report 69 centers in United States Funding Source: NHLBI	Registered cases of destination therapy	n=385 Mean Age (yr): 62 Male: 84% White: 76% Contraindications for Heart Transplant Age: 33% Renal: 22% Obesity: 16% Pulmonary: 20% Preop Profile: Shock: 9% Declining: 41% Inotrope: 26% Recurrent: 15%	HeartMate II (HMII) continuous flow LVAD (n=281) HeartMate XVE (HMXVE) pulsatile flow LVAD (n=104)	Actuarial Survival HMII HMXVE Month 3 86% 83% Month 6 81% 70% Month 12 74% 61% Month 24 na 39% p=0.02 (censored at transplant or device removal)	Not Randomized Baseline similarity not reported Different time periods No adjustments Not blinded Losses to follow-up not reported Intention to Treat (ITT) analysis Adequate number and precision of estimates
Strüber 2008[24] 12 centers in Europe Funding Source: Not reported	Consecutive cases; selection of patients for destination therapy not described	n= 31 Mean age (yr): 52 Otherwise not described	HeartMate II continuous flow LVAD used as destination therapy No control group	80% 3-month survival 71% 6-month survival 71% 1-year survival Other outcomes not reported for destination therapy subgroup	Small retrospective unblinded case series without a control group or description of baseline characteristics or follow-up

NYHA - New York Heart Association, IABP – intra-aortic balloon pump, IV – intravenous, ICD - implanted cardiac defibrillator, CRT - cardiac resynchronization therapy, LVAD - left ventricular assist device, HR – hazard ratio, CI - confidence interval, LHFQ - Minnesota Living with Heart Failure Questionnaire with lower scores indicating the patients perceived less adverse effects of heart failure on their quality of life, KCCQ - Kansas City Cardiomyopathy Questionnaire - the clinical score is a measure of physical function and heart failure symptoms with higher scores indicating less symptoms and better function

Use of Left Ventricular Assist Devices as Destination Therapy in End-Stage Congestive Heart Failure: A Systematic Review

Table 2. Key Question #2: Patient Selection

Study/Country/ Funding Source	Inclusion/Exclusion Criteria	Sample of Patients	Outcomes & Baseline Correlates	Study Quality

Kirklin 2011[3]
 	
69 centers in U.S.
 	
Funding Source: NIH, others
	Inclusion Criteria: Case registered in INTERMACS
	
	FDA-approved ventricular assist device implanted as destination therapy from June, 2006 to September 2010
		n = 385
		HeartMate II (n=281, 73%)
		HeartMate XVE (n=104, 27%)
		
		Mean Age (yr): 62
		Male: 84%
		White: 76%
		Black: 18%
		
		INTERMACS CLASSIFICATION
		Cardiogenic shock: 9%
		Progressive decline: 41%
		Inotrope dependent: 26%
		Recurrent decompensated heart failure: 15%
		Greatly limited exertion: 7%
		Class IIIb: 2%
		
		REASONS NOT ELIGIBLE FOR HEART TRANSPLANT
		Advanced age: 33%
		Renal dysfunction: 22%
		High body mass index: 16%
		Pulmonary hypertension: 12%
		Other: 17%
			Unspecified number and names of variables tested; reference groups for HR's are the complements of those described
			
			1) All-cause death within 30 days, n=35
			  a) cardiogenic shock
			    HR = 3.5, $p<0.01$
			  b) need for concomitant surgery
			    HR = 3.0, $p=0.02$
			  c) 10 units higher BUN
			    HR = 1.3, $p=0.001$
			
			2) All-cause deaths after 30 days, n=62
			  a) HeartMate XVE vs HeartMate II
			    HR = 2.75, $p=0.002$
			    interactions with other predictors not reported
			  b) pulmonary hypertension
			    HR = 3.6, $p=0.0001$
			  c) 10 units lower sodium
			    HR = 2.1, $p=0.005$
			  d) diabetes
			    HR = 2.0, $p=0.01$
			  e) age 70 vs 60 years
			    HR = 1.8, $p<0.0001$
				Patients eligible for destination therapy, but not all received HeartMate II
				
				Most variables assessed before implantation surgery
				
				Measurements of potential predictors not standardized or described
				
				Presumably complete follow-up of deaths
				
				Most predicted probabilities and confidence intervals not reported, no calibration or validation of prediction model
				
				No assessment of whether or how much use of variables could improve patient selection or outcomes

Levy 2009[33] 20 centers in U.S. Funding Source: Thoratec Corp	Inclusion Criteria Participants in clinical trial of HeartMate VE for destination therapy compared to optimal medical therapy (REMATCH Study)	n=129 (some missing values needed for the prediction model were imputed and use of inotropes or an intra-aortic balloon pump and/or ventilator were added to the prediction model) n= 61 in medical therapy arm Mean Age (yr): 67 Male: 80% Mean LVEF: 17% NYHA class IV: 100% IV inotrope: 56% Intra-aortic balloon pump: 8% Defibrillator: 35%	Survival predictions made using variables in the Seattle Heart Failure Model Average estimated 1-YEAR SURVIVAL in medical therapy arm (n = 37 deaths) 30% vs 28% observed 81% had < 50% estimated 1-year survival Note: guidelines for destination therapy recommend patient's expected 1-year survival be < 50% Interaction between treatment effect (assist device versus medical therapy) and Seattle Heart Failure Score was not significant ($p=0.86$)	Patients eligible for destination therapy, but none received HeartMate II Variables assessed before implantation surgery Measurements of potential predictors not standardized or described Complete follow-up for deaths No confidence intervals on predicted probabilities in small groups, a little information about calibration and validity of predictions Little assessment of whether or how much use of variables could improve patient selection or outcomes No evidence risk score discriminates groups of patients that do or do not have a survival benefit

Use of Left Ventricular Assist Devices as Destination Therapy in End-Stage Congestive Heart Failure: A Systematic Review

Study/Country/ Funding Source	Inclusion/Exclusion Criteria	Sample of Patients	Outcomes & Baseline Correlates	Study Quality
Lietz 2007[11] 56 centers in U.S. Funding Source: not reported	Inclusion Criteria Use of HeartMate XVE for destination therapy after FDA approval, November 2002 – 2005 Consent to be in manufacturer's case registry 280/309 (91%)	n= 280 (222 with complete data for analysis of in-hospital mortality) Mean Age (yr): 61 Male: 82% Mean LVEF: 18% IV inotrope: 70% NYHA class IV: 100%	Numerous variables examined by stepwise logistic regression including demographics and body size, cause of heart failure, history of cardiovascular diseases, other comorbidities, medical and device therapy for heart failure, hemodynamics, laboratory data, year and center experience. Regression estimates used to calculate individual risk score. 90-DAY IN-HOSPITAL MORTALITY, n=60 (27%) CAUSES Sepsis - 33% Multiorgan failure - 20% Right heart failure - 14% Respiratory failure - 7% Technical difficulties - 5% Device failure - 5% Hemorrhage - 3% Stroke - 3% Several other causes - 10% INDEPENDENT CORRELATES (OR = odds ratio) Platelet count $\leq$ 148,000; OR = 7.7 Serum albumin $\leq$ 3.3 g/dl; OR = 5.7 INR > 1.1; OR = 5.4 Vasodilator; OR = 5.2 Mean pulmonary artery pressure $\leq$ 25 mmHg; OR = 4.1 Aspartate aminotransferase > 45 U/ml; OR = 2.6 Hematocrit $\leq$ 34%; OR = 3.0 Blood urea nitrogen > 51 U/dl; OR = 2.9 No IV inotrope; OR = 2.9	Patients eligible for destination therapy, but none received HeartMate II Variables assessed before implantation surgery Measurements of potential predictors not standardized or described Presumably complete follow-up of in-hospital deaths Wide confidence intervals on predicted probabilities, calibration questionable, and predictions not validated No assessment of whether or how much use of variables could improve patient selection or outcomes; thresholds of acceptable operative risk not defined

Use of Left Ventricular Assist Devices as Destination Therapy in End-Stage Congestive Heart Failure: A Systematic Review

Evidence-based Synthesis Program

Study/Country/ Funding Source	Inclusion/Exclusion Criteria	Sample of Patients	Outcomes & Baseline Correlates	Study Quality
Leitz 2007[11] Continued	See above	See above	RISK SCORE C-statistic 0.89 RISK SCORE CATEGORIES % PREDICTED (CI) vs OBS 0 to 8 (n=65) 2 (1 to 5) vs 6 9 to 16 (n=111) 12 (8 to 18) vs 14 17 to 19 (n=28) 44 (33 to 56) vs 61 >19 (n=18) 81 (66 to 91) vs 82	See above

Adamson 2011[34]
 	
Single center in U.S.
 	
Funding Source: not reported
	Inclusion Criteria
	Patients enrolled in clinical trials of the HeartMate II ventricular assist device
	
	All carefully screened using criteria of clinical trials and CMS
		n=55 subgrouped into <70 (n=25) and ≥70 years old (n=30)
		
		Male: not reported
		NYHA class IV: 100%
		Mean LVEF: 20%
		IV inotrope: 64%
		Intra-aortic balloon pump: 5%
		Defibrillator: 74%
		Cardiac resynchronization therapy: 51%
		Mean Destination Therapy Risk Score: 9.3
			<70 group ≥70 group
			MEAN AGE (years) 57 76
			MEDIAN DURATION WITH DEVICE (days)
			                415 482
			DROPOUTS 3 0
			SURVIVAL (p=0.81)
			30 days 96% 97%
			6 months 88% 83%
			12 months 72% 75%
			AT 6 MONTHS
			NYHA CLASS I or II 100% 89% p=0.35
			MEAN IMPROVE in MLHFQ SCORE
			                36 42 p=0.07
			MEAN IMPROVE in KCCQ SCORE
			                32 42 p=0.88
			
			ADVERSE EVENT RATES
			No significant differences
			Major Bleeding 28% 30%
			Sepsis 24% 20%
			Device-related infect. 20% 17%
			Cardiac Arrhythmia 32% 33%
			Stroke 8% 10%
			Right heart failure 4% 3%
			Renal failure 4% 3%
				Patients eligible for destination therapy, received HeartMate II
				
				Age determined before implantation surgery and likely valid
				
				Presumably complete follow-up in trials
				
				No confidence intervals on differences between small age subgroups
				
				No adjustment for preoperative differences

INTERMACS – Interagency Registry for Mechanically Assisted Circulatory Support, LVEF – left ventricular ejection fraction, IV – intravenous, NYHA – New York Heart Association, HR – hazard ratio, OR – odds ratio, INR – international normalization ratio, CI – 95% confidence interval, OBS – observed, BUN – blood urea nitrogen, MLHFQ – Minnesota Living with Heart Failure Score, KCCQ – Kansas City Cardiomyopathy Questionnaire

Use of Left Ventricular Assist Devices as Destination Therapy in End-Stage Congestive Heart Failure: A Systematic Review

Table 3. Key Question #3: Cost-effectiveness

Study/Design/ Funding Source	Key Model Components and Source	Base Case	Sensitivity Analyses	Range in ICER per QALY*	Study Limitations
Rogers 2012[35] Cost-effectiveness analysis of continuous-flow LVAD versus OMM using a Markov model Funding Source: Thoratec Corp	24-mo survival for LVAD[1]	KM curve	NA	NA	The data regarding the difference in the effect of LVAD vs. OMM involves an indirect comparison across 2 RCTs
	24-mo survival for OMM[2]	KM curve	NA	NA	
	Long-term survival extrapolation for LVAD[3]	Exponential	Linear, Stop and drop	$180,000-$375,000	
	Long-term survival extrapolation for OMM[3]	Exponential	NA	$150,000-$250,000	The long-term outcome data are extrapolated from 2 years of RCT data
	LVAD implantation hospital cost[4]	$193,812	$122,785–$264,839	NA	
	LVAD implantation professional service cost[5]	$8,841	NA	NA	
	LVAD replacement cost[6]	$131,430	NA	NA	All sensitivity analyses only varied one parameter at a time, whereas a probabilistic model that allows multiple parameters to vary at the same time might more accurately assess the overall uncertainty in the model
	Monthly LVAD replacement rate[1]	0.005	NA	NA	
	Rehospitalization cost (per event)[7,8]	$6,850	$6,850–$30,627	$200,000-$280,000	
	Monthly rehospitalization rate for LVAD[1]	0.21	NA	NA	
	Monthly rehospitalization rate for OMM[7]	0.1325	0.1325-0.26	$195,000-$200,000	
	Monthly outpatient costs[9,10]	$2,331	NA	NA	
	End-of-life cost[11]	$44,211	NA	NA	
	Utility for NYHA Class I[12]	0.855	0.641-1.0	$180,000-$230,000	Utilities used to calculate quality-adjusted life years were based on NYHA classes
	Utility for NYHA Class II[12]	0.771	0.578-0.964	$175,000-$225,000	
	Utility for NYHA Class III[12]	0.673	0.505-0.841	$190,000-$205,000	
	Utility for NYHA Class IV[12]	0.532	0.399-0.665	$190,000-$200,000	

LVAD – left ventricular assist device, OMM – optimal medical management, NYHA – New York Heart Association, RCT – randomized controlled trial, ICER – incremental cost-effectiveness ratio, QALY- quality adjusted life year

*This is the range in Incremental Cost Effectiveness Ratio per Quality Adjusted Life Year when the model is varied over the range of values in the sensitivity analysis. The values were roughly estimated to approximately the nearest $5,000 using Figure 3 from Rogers et al., 2012.[35]

Table 3. Reference List

(1) Slaughter MS, Rogers JG, Milano CA, Russell SD, Conte JV, Feldman D et al. Advanced heart failure treated with continuous-flow left ventricular assist device. *N Engl J Med.* 2009;361(23):2241-51.

(2) Rose EA, Gelijns AC, Moskowitz AJ, Heitjan DF, Stevenson LW, Dembitsky W et al. Long-term use of a left ventricular assist device for end-stage heart failure. *N Engl J Med.* 2001;345(20):1435-43.

(3) Special report: cost-effectiveness of left-ventricular assist devices as destination therapy for end-stage heart failure. *Technol Eval Cent Asses Program Exec Summ* 2004 April;19(2):1.

(4) Slaughter MS, Bostic R, Tong K, Russo M, Rogers JG. Temporal changes in hospital costs for left ventricular assist device implantation. *J Card Surg.* 2011;26(5):535-41.

(5) Centers for Medicare and Medicaid Services.Standard Analytic File, 2008. Centers for Medicare and Medicaid Services, Baltimore, MD.

(6) Medicare Program; changes to the hospital inpatient prospective payment systems and fiscal year 2009 rates; payments for graduate medical education in certain emergency situations; changes to disclosure of physician ownership in hospitals and physician self-referral rules; updates to the long-term care prospective payment system; updates to certain IPPS-excluded hospitals; and collection of information regarding financial relationships between hospitals; final rule. *Federal Register.* 73;8-19-2008.

(7) Anand IS, Carson P, Galle E, Song R, Boehmer J, Ghali JK et al. Cardiac resynchronization therapy reduces the risk of hospitalizations in patients with advanced heart failure: results from the Comparison of Medical Therapy, Pacing and Defibrillation in Heart Failure (COMPANION) trial. *Circulation.* 2009;119(7):969-77.

(8) Oz MC, Gelijns AC. Miller L, Wang C, Nickens P, Arons R et al. Left ventricular assist devices as permanent heart failure therapy: the price of progress. *Ann Surg.* 2003;238(4):577-83.

(9) Gelijns AC, Richards AF, Williams DL, Oz MC, Oliveira J, Moskowitz AJ. Evolving costs of long-term left ventricular assist device implantation. *Ann Thorac Surg.* 1997;64(5):1312-9.

(10) Moskowitz AJ, Rose EA, Gelijns AC. The cost of long-term LVAD implantation. *Ann Thorac Surg.* 2001;71(3 Suppl):S195-S198.

(11) Russo MJ, Gelijns AC, Stevenson LW, Sampat B, Aaronson KD, Renlund DG et al. The cost of medical management in advanced heart failure during the final two years of life. *J Card Fail.* 2008;14(8):651-8.

(12) Gohler A, Geisler EP, Manne JM, Kosiborod M, Zhang Z, Weintraub WS et al. Utility estimates for decision-analytic modeling in chronic heart failure—health states based on New York Heart Association classes and number of rehospitalizations. *Value Health* 2009;12(1):185-7.

www.ingramcontent.com/pod-product-compliance
Lightning Source LLC
Chambersburg PA
CBHW081359170526
45166CB00010B/3137